China's Traditional Way of Health Preservation

Zeng Qingnan
Liu Daoqing

FOREIGN LANGUAGES PRESS   BEIJING

First Edition 2002
Second Printing   2008

Home Page:
   http://www.flp.com.cn
E-mail Addresses:
   info@flp.com.cn
   sales@flp.com.cn

ISBN 978-7-119-02016-7

Published by Foreign Languages Press
24 Baiwanzhuang Road, Beijing 100037, China
Distributed by China International Book Trading Corporation
35 Chegongzhuang Xilu, Beijing 100044, China
P. O. Box 399, Beijing, China

Printed in the People's Republic of China

Contents

Introduction

Human Life Expectancy

All living things have a fairly fixed life expectancy. For example, a cat can live as long as 10 years, a dog 18 years, an ox 30 years, a horse 40 years, an elephant 150 years, a turtle 300 years and a whale 400 years. Then how long can a man live? Scientists have made a long and deep study of this question and found the following methods of calculation which conform to the law of life expectancy of man and animals: The life expectancy of mammals should be five to seven times their growth period. The human growth period is about 20-25 years. Calculated on this basis, the life expectancy limit of man should be 100 to 175 years. Wu Keqian, a Chinese physician during the Qing Dynasty(1644-1911), wrote in his book *Instructions on Health Building ·Preface*: "From the time he is born, a man grows fully (matures) by the age of 25. In proportion to the length of the life of animals, man should live as long as 125 years or 200 years."

Calculating by the sexual maturity period, scientists have pointed out that the highest life expectancy for mammals is generally 8-10 times their sexual maturity period. The human sexual maturity period is generally 14-15 years. Calculated on this basis, the highest life expectancy of man should be 112 to 150 years.

Calculating by the number of times that cells divide, an American cytologist made a study of the law of the division and proliferation of cells of human embryo fibers and proposed methods for calculating human life expectancy based on the number of times that cells divide. The pulmonary fiber cells of the chicken are divided 13-35 times and its life expectancy is 30 years. The pulmonary fiber cells of the sea turtle are divided 72-114 times and its life expectancy is 300 years. The average cycle of the division of the pulmonary fiber cells of all animals is 2.4 years. The pulmonary fiber cells of human beings divide about 50 times. Calculated on this basis, the highest life expectancy limit for human beings should be 120 years.

Calculating by pregnancy, Ermonsky, a Soviet biologist, said there is a variation coefficient of embryo development and life expectancy of human beings, and it is 15.15. The human gestation period is 266 days. When this figure is multiplied by 15.15, it equals 11 years. If it is multiplied by 15.15 again, it should be 167 years. This is the highest limit of life expectancy for human beings.

Calculating by the viability of organs and tissues, experiments have proved that human organs and tissues can live many years outside the human body. If calculated on this basis, the tissues and organs of human beings can work for 140-150 years. It can thus be seen that the highest limit of human life expectancy can be 150 years.

Calculated on the basis of these theories, the top limit of human life expectancy should be over 100 years. Some people argue that it should be 120 years, some believe that it should be 150 years, some 180 years and some 200 years. Suharevsky of the former Soviet Union even argued that it should be 400 years.

In fact, there were people who lived to that age and longer. There are many records of this in ancient China. *The Incidents in the Reign of Kaiyuan* (713-742) in the Tang Dynasty says: "Yu Bolong in Taiyuan was still full of vigor when at the age of 128. His son had died, but his two grandsons of 70 and 80 years old lived with him. The book *The Annals of Dong Wei* says: "Yang Xiaju is several small parts, of the DNA. In other words, there are repetitions of these genes. The genes of species with long-life elements in their DNA molecules also have more gene reserves. As one ages, the DNA molecules are constantly damaged and the reserve genes are constantly used. When the reserve genes are completely consumed, old age comes. Other scholars hold that with increased age, more and more errors are made in the information transmission system, thus reducing the function of the cells and leading to old age. Still other scholars hold that there are "old age genes," and they are activated at a certain period of life, bringing about retrogressive changes in the organism. And the accumulation of these retrogressive changes leads to old age. How do the hereditary genes control old age? There is still no final answer at present. A definite conclusion will be made only after more research.

The theory of endocrinopathy. The endocrine system includes the sexual gland, the thoracic gland, the pituitary gland, the thyroid gland and the adrenal gland. The hormones they secrete are closely related to the growth, development and physiological functions of the human body. Therefore, these hormones can accelerate or delay the aging process. After middle age, the functions of the endocrine glands become gradually weak, leading to the gradual decline of their physiological function and therefore to old age.

The theory of immunity. Immunity is a physiological function of the human body. Depending on this function, the organism distinguishes itself from alien elements, and excludes and destroys the antigens (such as virus, bacteria and tumor cells) that have invaded the organism, or the isomeric substances (such as dead and damaged cells) produced by the organism itself. Immunity protects the human body by resisting bacterial infection, but on the other hand, it can be detrimental in such cases as allergy, autoimmunity and transplantation immunity. For example, when a patient with extensive burns needs skin grafting, apart from grafting the healthy skin from his own body, the skin from others is also used. However, the grafted skin is vulnerable to necrosis. This is exactly the immune function of excluding alien elements. The immunity of the human body originates with the lymphocytes. Lymphocytes are divided into two categories: One category originates from the B cells in the marrow, and the other from the T cells in the thoracic glands. The lymphocytes can identify and destroy the alien elements such as bacteria, viruses, fungus, cancer cells and poisonous substances, thus protecting the organism. After middle age, the thoracic gland declines (it is 40 grams in puberty, and is reduced to 10 grams by old age), the reproduction of the T cells slows down, and the quantity decreases. The normal immunity of the B cells also becomes weak, thus increasing the incidence of malignant tumors and other diseases of old age. At the same time, the lymphocytes in middle-aged and old people seem to lose some of their identifying ability. They then fail to distinguish the invading cells from the body's own cells, with the result that their own cells are also destroyed. This is called "autoimmunity." The increase of the reaction of "autoimmunity" leads to the increase of the diseases of autoimmunity such as rheumatoid arthritis, thus accelerating the aging process.

The theory of the central nervous system. Under normal conditions, from the time a man is born until the age of 50, the weight of his cerebrum increases gradually. This increase in the weight of the cerebrum is fastest between ages 6 and 10. It becomes obviously slower between ages 21 and 30, and declines after 60. As the cerebrum cortex maintains the normal functions of the human body through the central nerve and its surrounding nervous system, whether the central nerve cells decline or not plays an extremely important role in the aging process. Experiments have shown that the tension of the cerebrum cortex and the imbalance of the internal and external surroundings of the human body weaken the functions of the internal organs in the whole body. The more developed the cerebrum, the longer the life span. The decline of the cerebrum gives rise to the early aging.

The theory of autointoxication. As the function of the excretory organs declines, the products of metabolism, such as phenol, indole and pigments, are apt to deposit in and intoxicate the cells. If more and more of these poisonous substances are deposited in the cells and the cells beome intoxicated, they decline and eventually die. As a result, the internal organs and the human body become old and weak.

The knowledge of the cause of old age in traditional Chinese medicine. Traditional Chinese medicine attributes life-span and health to the function of the kidneys. The kidneys are "the foundation of the innate" and the "chief commander." They command reproduction and thinking. The functions of the kidneys include some of the functions of the reproductive system, the endocrine system, the central nervous system, and the immunity system. A man with the strong sap of the kidneys is not only full of vigor and quick-minded, he also enjoys good health and has a longer life. This ancient knowledge also holds that aging is closely related to the living environment and habits. For example, *The Yellow Emperor's Canon of Medicine,* holds that people living in cold and high mountainous regions have a longer life, while those living in damp, hot, and low-lying regions have a shorter life. It also says: "People in remote ages followed the law of Yin and Yang, were reconciled to magical calculations and fortune-telling, controlled their diets, and lived a regulated life. They did not overwork themselves, so they had sound bodies and minds and lived to the age of 100. The people of today do the opposite. They drink wine like water, often wildly, and have sex when they are drunk in order to exhaust their energy and consume their vitality.

They do not know how to feel satisfied or protect their energy, but only seek sensuous pleasures. Since they ignore the laws for proper living and live without restraint, they may die at 50." This passage deals with the relationship between the aging process and living habits. It means that as long as you are moderate in eating and drinking, have a regular life and do not overwork yourself, you will enjoy good health and have a long life. Otherwise, you may become old and weak by the age of 50.

Chapter One

Seasonal Methods

Man lives in nature, and his existence and health are necessarily affected by the natural environment. A good natural environment is undoubtedly beneficial to a tranquil mind, good health and long life.

Traditional Chinese medicine holds that the human body is a "small world." This "small world" is linked to the large world of nature. In other words, the movements of the large world such as the movement of the celestial bodies, sunspots activity, the changes of weather in the four seasons, and changes in geographical surroundings all affect the "small world" of the human body. That is, the physiological activities of the human body are directly affected by cosmic movement. If the human body can accommodate itself to the changes in its natural surroundings, it can exist healthily. Otherwise, it is vulnerable to diseases and life may be threatened.

The natural environment may be divided into climate and geography. Generally, people living in cold mountainous regions with fresh air have a longer life than those living in hot regions with fouler air. In cold climates, living things have a longer growth period and therefore have a longer life, while in hot regions living things have a shorter growth period and therefore have a shorter life.

When this is understood, man can on his own initiative protect the natural environment on which he depends for survival, accommodate himself to natural changes, or even transform the natural environment to make it better suited for the existence of mankind.

The four seasons change each year, and the day changes from morning to evening, from day to night. How should people accommodate themselves to the change of seasons and the changes of the day to promote good health?

1. Spring

In spring, the weather becomes warmer, the ice melts and the snow thaws, the land comes back to life and all the plants turn green. The hibernating animals wake up, the willows bud and the flowers bloom. The natural world is alive again with vigor. As it continues to get warmer, the skin begins to stretch, and the functional activities of the internal organs, vital energy and blood increase. In this season, how is health best preserved?

Conform to springtime. When the natural world is full of life, man should also exert himself to arouse the vitality within his body so that the small world of the human body and the large world of nature are both filled with the vigor of spring, and the external and internal environments complement each other. Get up early in the morning and take a carefree walk in the courtyard or in the park or in the greenery along the road, stretch the four limbs and the whole body as much as possible, and open the mind to everything, without restraint.

Take spring trips from time to time. The sun is bright, the birds sing, the flowers give forth their fragrance, the peach trees are in red, the willows are turning green, and the wheat fields are also becoming green. The beautiful scenes of the natural world are fascinating and intoxicating. Going to the scenic spots and into the hills not only helps mold your temperament and open your mind, but also broadens your horizon, invigorates your blood circulation, regulates your nervous system, and improves the soundness of body and mind.

Protection against spring cold. There is an old saying in China: "Get more clad in spring and less clad in autumn." In other words, don't take off your winter clothes too early in spring. It is better to feel a little warmer than to feel cold. Clothes should be shed gradually as the weather gets warmer to enable the body to adapt gradually to the warmer weather. Conversely, one should not put on winter clothes too soon in autumn, it is better to feel a bit colder than to feel too hot. This enables the body to adapt gradually to the colder weather. One becomes less vulnerable to illness in this way. Spring is the transitional season between winter and summer, when the weather changes from cold to warm. If people do not take care to keep themselves warm and instead take off their winter clothes too early, they catch cold easily, and the patients with high blood pressure may even suffer cerebral hemorrhage. Therefore, one must take special care during the seasonal changes to guard against the cold and keep warm.

Preventing the common cold. Many people catch cold three times a year. Middle-aged and older people in poor health may catch cold even more often. Spring is the season when people catch cold most easily. Why? There are two main reasons. One is the abrupt change in the temperature in spring when people may take off their winter clothes too soon as the weather becomes suddenly warmer. When attacked by the cold, resistance drops and the immunity function becomes weak, so people catch cold more easily. The second reason is the strong spring wind when the pathogenic bacteria and viruses in the air move easily to cause diseases of the respiratory system. Some middle-aged and older people also are apt to suffer from infectious diseases of the upper respiratory tract if they are physically weak and fail to heed the changing weather. These people should take special care to guard against the cold and keep themselves warm. Moreover, they should make an effort to train themselves against the cold. For example, using cold wet towels to wash their face and cold water to rinse their throat helps to increase their ability to resist the cold. They should regularly massage the Yingxiang, Hegu, Quchi and Fengchi acupoints (see appendix). This also helps to keep you fit and healthy. When cold prevails, boil cooking vinegar and use its steam to sterilize the house. Or decoct rhizome of cyrtomium (15 grams) and honeysuckle (20 grams) and take orally, one dose a day for three days. These methods all help to prevent cold and the recurrence of old illnesses. As the weather changes abruptly in spring, the masculine energy in the liver rises. If more heat is accumulated in the body, it easily leads to the recurrence of an old illness in middle-aged and older people, such as acute and chronic bronchitis, the abrupt rise of blood pressure in people with hypertension, aggravated symptoms from agitated activity, weary limbs, insomnia and dizziness. Be sure to keep physically fit and prevent the recurrence of old illnesses in accordance with weather changes in the spring.

2. Summer

The weather is hot in summer, the yang *qi* (masculine energy) is strong, and blood vessels throughout the body dilate. Both *qi* (vital energy) and blood flow to the body surface, and it is easy to perspire, causing listlessness and a poor appetite. Therefore it is very important to build your health in summer. How?

Adapt yourself to summertime. All things grow luxuriantly, the essence from heaven falls while that from the earth rises. When the two essences meet, all things blossom and bear fruit. People should go to bed late and rise early. Do not dislike the long day and hot weather, but do more things outdoors so as to become relaxed and happy instead of agitated. This is the rule for good health in summer.

Mental cultivation. In the hot summer, middle-aged and older people should pay attention to mental cultivation. As long as they keep calm and have peace of mind, they will feel cool and get rid of the heat. An old saying goes: "One does not feel the heat too much as long as one keeps calm." This is the best way to keep fit and prevent heat stroke.

Do not be too greedy for coolness. Old people are deficient both in the *qi* and blood. As the pores all open in the hot summer, heat and sweat comes out, and they become vulnerable to an attack of the cold air, causing wandering arthritis such as pain in the joints, insensitivity and paralysis of limbs. Therefore, middle-aged and older people must take preventive measures to reduce the heat and be sure not to be greedy for coolness. Do not sleep on the damp floor, in the passageway, or under the eaves, nor use an electric fan when you sleep so as to avoid attacks of cold pathogens which may cause such diseases as deviation of the eye and mouth and hemiplegia. An old Chinese folk saying goes: "Take shelter from the wind just like the arrows. If you are avaricious for the cool air when you sleep, illness goes with you." All these are valuable examples of the experience accumulated from long practice, and they are worth following to build your health in summer.

If you fall asleep as you enjoy the cool, you should use a towel to cover your navel and abdomen, because the navel is vulnerable to cold. Once you become cold, your digestive function is affected causing stomach ache or loose bowels and disorders of the digestive system.

Build health through food. The diet of middle-aged and older people in summer should consist of light and digestible food such as vegetables, beans, fruits, melons and porridges. Watermelon is refreshing in the summer heat. It is nutritious and helps make the loss of water and dielectric caused by sweating. It is hot in summer, but one should not take too much cold food so as to avoid functional disorders of the intestines and stomach leading to stomachache, vomiting and loose bowels. Be sure not to eat spoiled food polluted by bacteria to avoid infectious diseases of the digestive tract such as enteritis and dysentery.

Preventing heat disorders. When one works in a hot environment the heat generated inside the body does not spread quickly, and the gradual rise in body temperature may cause headache, nausea, weakness in the limbs, and even fainting. This is heatstroke. When one works or walks in the very hot sun, the dilation of the cerebral blood vessels and encephalemia may cause headache, dizziness, or unconsciousness. This is sunstroke. The body keeps sweating under the excessive heat and the water content and dielectric in the body drop greatly, causing dizziness, thirst, irritation, tics and sore muscles. This is heat spasms. All these disorders are caused by hot temperatures. They may also be caused by wind velocity, intense labor, long exposure to the sun, weak physical condition, inadequate nutrition, deficiency of water and salt, and general health condition. When the average day temperature is higher than 31 degrees Centigrade, the number of people affected by the heat increases markedly. When the temperature exceeds 37 degrees Centigrade for several days, the number of people who suffer from excessive heat rises radically. When the temperature is very hot in summer, labor intensity should be reduced. When working in the fields or walking outside, one should use an umbrella or a hat, wear white or light color clothes, and rest in the shade or in places with cool air. Get plenty of sleep. If one sweats too much, eat watermelon and take cold drinks. There are some of the drinks used by Chinese people to prevent heat and sun disorders:

Honeysuckle (or chrysanthemum) 30 g, water 1,500 ml, boil

for 5 minutes, cool the liquid, and drink anytime.

Mung beans (or red beans) 200 g, sugar 30 g, water 3,000 ml, boil for 1 hour, cool the liquid, and drink anytime.

Fresh plums 60 g, ice sugar 30 g, water 1,000 ml, boil for 1 hour, cool the liquid and drink anytime.

These drinks not only help you cool down, they also help increase urination, stimulate the heart, and reduce blood pressure. So they are good for people suffering from hypertension, heart trouble, and urinary tract infections.

If you travel, take some heat-preventing drugs with you, such as the 10 drops, rendan, Huoxiang Zhengqi Shui (liquid of agastache for restoring health), cooling ointment, and essential balm.

3. Autumn

The weather gets cool gradually in autumn, solar energy decreases day by day while lunar energy increases. The scene becomes desolate. In the life process of "coming into being, growth, maturity, retreat and hiding" autumn belongs to the period of retreat. The word "retreat" has dual implications: One is "harvest," that is, the crops ripen and the trees and grass bear fruit and seed, and it is time to harvest. The other is "withdrawal," that is, when the autumn wind soughs, all things transform from the stage of vigorous growth to the stage of "retreat," and there is a desolate sight everywhere. How can you build health in this season?

Adapt to the autumn season. The weather changes from hot to cool and all things retreat. The life of the people should be adapted to the autumn. Go to sleep early and rise early, withdraw vigor, do not tax yourself too much and keep peace of mind to alleviate the influence of the autumn desolation on your body.

Do not wear too many clothes too soon, or dress too warmly. It is better to be cool than to be over-dressed. As the old saying goes: "Get more clad in spring and less in autumn." To be less clad in autumn helps to adapt the body gradually to the cold weather, and increases the body's resistance.

Adjust your diet. In autumn, attention should be paid to moistening the dryness and nourishing the kidneys and lungs. More sesame seeds, honey, milk, fresh fruits and vegetables should be eaten for this purpose. As the digestive functions of middle-aged and older people become weak gradually, it is advisable to eat porridge for breakfast and supper. Use glutinous rice 50 g and fresh Chinese yam 30 g to make the porridge. This helps nourish the stomach and makes it less dry in autumn. It is a good food for middle-aged and old people in autumn.

Nourishment from medicine. The weather changes capriciously. Sometimes it is very hot and sometimes very cold, and the temperature difference is big between day and night during the period between the two solar terms of the Beginning of Autumn (August 7) and the Beginning of Winter (November 7). This can easily cause illness. In order to prevent illness and balance Yin and Yang, it is necessary to get some nourishment from drugs. The major principles for nourishment from drugs are: one, nourish the feminine energy and alleviate dryness, and two, improve the spleen and stomach to prevent the desolateness from harming the body as well as to prevent stomachache and loose bowels that might result from overeating raw and cold melons and fruits. To nourish feminine energy and alleviate dryness, it is advisable to use Dangshen (Asiabell root) 6 g, uncooked yam 10 g, Maidong (lilyturf roots) 6 g, honey 6 g and pears 15 g and decoct them with water. Or eat porridge cooked with Shengdi dried (rehmannia roots), porridge with Chinese yam, porridge cooked with Maidong (lilyturf roots) or porridge with Baihe (lily). Here is how to make them:

Porridge with dried rehmannia roots: dried rehmannia root 10 g, lotus seeds 10 g, round-grained non-glutinous rice 20 g and water 500 ml. Boil in water over low fire for 40 minutes.

Porridge with Chinese yam: fresh yam 30 g (or powdered yam 10 g), round- grained non-glutinous rice 30 g, and water 500 ml. Make it the same way.

Porridge with lilyturf roots: lilyturf roots 10 g, round-grained non-glutinous rice 30 g, and water 500 ml. Make it the same way.

Porridge with lily: fresh lily 20 g (or dried lily 10 g), round-grained non-glutinous rice 30 g, and water 500 ml. Make it the same way.

To improve the spleen and stomach and nourish the vital energy, it is advisable to use Huoxiang (giant hyssop) 6 g, haws stir-fried over fire 6 g, white hyacinth beans stir-fried over fire 10 g, 5 large dates, Yiyiren (Job's tears seed) 10 g, Yunling (Indian bread from Yunnan) 10 g and dried tangerine peels 4 g. Decoct them in water, and take the decoction once a week.

4. Winter

Winter is the coldest season of the year. In the life process, winter is the "hiding" season. How can people maintain health in this season?

Adapt to the wintertime. So far as human activities are concerned, people should hide "the semen," " the mind" and "the body." "Hiding the semen" means conserving the semen and storing up energy for "budding" the next spring. Concretely speaking, be moderate in sex to avoid losing too much semen. At the same time, avoid excessive physical work and physical exercise, because this will cause too much sweating and harm the semen and masculine energy. "Hiding the mind" means not overtaxing the mind but reducing thinking as if to hide consciousness. "Hiding the body" means keeping oneself in doors. Do as little outdoors as possible to keep oneself away from an attack of cold which says *qi* (vital energy) and causes illness. Keep the house warm, go to bed early and rise late. It is best to get up when the sun rises.

In the long-time practice of health protection, the health builders have founded the theory of "nourishing the masculine energy in spring and summer, and nourishing the Yin *qi* (feminine energy) in autumn and winter." "Nourishing the masculine energy in spring and summer" means doing more outdoors and physical exercise in spring and summer to build up a good physique and refresh the body and mind in nature, full of vitality (masculine energy). "Nourishing the Yin *qi* in autumn and winter" means reducing physical exercises, withdrawing and hiding consciousness, and controlling sex in order to store up the Yin *qi*.

Nourishing food in winter. As both the vital energy and blood of middle-aged and old people decline, it is necessary that they have proper nourishment. Nourishment includes both drugs and food. Drug nourishment means taking drugs orally to improve vital energy, blood and semen. Food nourishment means eating the proper food to nourish the kidneys and generate the semen, invigorate the heart and spleen, improve the functions of the lungs, and promote the secretion of salvia and body fluids. Since it is cold in winter, it is advisable that middle-aged and old people take some nourishment. First of all, we will touch on food nourishment.

Nutritious foods that should be taken by middle-aged and older people in winter are those with both mild and hot properties, such as mutton and rabbit meat. They have hot properties and are good for strengthening the kidneys and building up the semen and blood. Chicken and fish have mild properties and are good for building up *qi* (vital energy), and promoting the generation of semen and marrow. Also, shrimp, sea cucumber, hen eggs, fungus, soy beans, Chinese yam, millet, large dates, walnuts, and bee honey are all good and nutritious foods.

Following are some nutritious foods which were commonly used for middle-aged and older people in winter in ancient times. Apart from nourishing the organs, improving the physique and prolonging the life, they are also good for curing senile diseases:

Walnut kernels 15 g, honey 30 g, sweet almonds 15 g. Steam in a bowl until they are done, and add five drops of ginger extract. Take it separately on two occasions, to cure the dry cough without phlegm in old people.

One crucian carp. Remove the scales and internal organs, wash clean, mince the meat, add some shredded ginger, and braise it with flavorings. It helps cure stomachache.

Pork cooked with chestnuts is a good cure for loose bowels.

One carp about 500 g. Remove the scales and internal organs, add small red beans 15g, wax gourd 250 g, onion whites 5 pieces. Cook them in water without salt. Eat the fish, drink the soup, and sleep with a coverlet for slight sweating. This is good for nourishing the kidneys, strengthening the spleen, and warming Yang (vital function) to induce diuresis. It is a good cure for dropsy and nephritis.

Stir-fried Chinese yam 30 g, stir-fried Job's tears seeds 30 g, lotus seeds 30 g and stir-fried white hyacinth beans 10 g. Powder them and cook them with six large dates. This is good for improving the spleen and diarrhea.

Water chestnuts 30 g, and large dates with the pits removed 30 g. Cook with water and eat twice a day. This is a cure for blood in stool.

Dried longan pulp, lotus seeds and large dates with the pits removed, 15 g each. Cook in water. Eat twice a day. It is good for palpitations, insomnia and amnesia.

Lotus seeds 15 g, and dried long an pulp 15 g, lily 10 g, yam

10 g, three large dates with pits removed, round-grained non-glutinous rice 15 g. Cook in water and make into a porridge, eat twice a day. This is a good cure for insomnia, amnesia, palpitations, and deficiency of *qi* (vital energy) in both the heart and spleen.

Fresh Jicai (shepherd's purse) or fresh celery, without salt or a little salt. Eat it often. It is good for hypertension.

Prawns 60 g. Fry in sesame oil until well done. Chives 100 g. Wash clean and stir-fry. Eat them together, they are good for strengthening the kidneys, and good cure for impotence and premature ejaculation.

Stem heads of celery 250 g. Crush to extract the juice, add sugar (or ice sugar) 10 g, mix them and drink it when cool. Or use celery 250 g and 10 large dates, and boil them in water for oral use. This nourishes the kidneys and improves the liver. It also cures hypertension and headache.

Dried Chinese yam. Powder and cook, 30 g each time, with rice porridge and eat twice a day. Take it for six months without stopping, it is good for diabetes.

Burnt Huangqi (milkvetch roots) 15 g, ginseng 6 g, round-grained non-glutinous rice 30 g, and sugar 10 g. First soak the milkvetch root and ginseng in water for 30 minutes, and then boil them in an earthenware pot for 1 hour. Remove the residue, and add the sugar and rice to make porridge. Take orally. This helps resist aging, improves the functions of the spleen and stomach, increases vital energy, and makes up for deficiency.

Heshouwu (fleeceflower root) 30 g, round-grained non-glutinous rice 30 g, 5 red dates, and a proper amount of brown sugar. First decoct the fleeceflower root into thick soup, and then add the other ingredients to make porridge. This helps cure early greying of the hair, reduce fat in the blood, and resist aging.

Shanyurou (dogwood fruit) 15 g, round-grained non-glutinous

rice 30 g and a proper amount of sugar. Cook with water into a porridge. This helps nourish the kidneys, increase semen, and cure dizziness, tinnitus, mental fatigue and physical weakness.

Roucongrong (cistanche) 10 g, lean mutton 30 g and round-grained non-glutinous rice 30 g. First decoct the cistanche for 1 hour and remove the liquid. Mince the mutton, add the rice and water, and cook together with the saline cistanche liquid to make porridge. When ready, add a proper amount of refined salt, shredded ginger and onion white. This helps cure deficiency of the Yang *qi* (masculine energy) in the spleen and kidneys, impotence and premature ejaculation, and lumbago and sore knees.

All these nutritious foods can be eaten regularly. Change your diet from time to time and increase food variety as much as possible so your body will get all kinds of nutriment. Be sure not to eat one food too much, as this may harm your spleen and stomach. Moreover, most nutritious foods have a hot or warm property. If you eat too much, they may cause an accumulation of internal heat resulting in headache, toothache and sore throat.

Medicinal nutrition in winter. By taking nutritious medicines in winter, middle-aged and older people can make up for deficiencies, cure illnesses, prolong life, and stay healthy. Some common nutritious medicines for these people are discussed as follows.

Traditional Chinese patent medicines for toning the kidneys and invigorating the masculine energy: Jinkui Shenqi Wan, Qiju Dihuang Wan, Shiquan Dabu Wan, Guilingji capsules and Shenrong tablets. These medicines are good for people who are affected by cold, physically weak people, and people of the cold-deficiency type.

Traditional Chinese patent medicines for nourishing the feminine energy to check an exuberance of the masculine energy: Zhibai Dihuang Wan, Maiwei Dihuang Wan, Liuwei Dihuang Wan, Qiongyu Ointment, and Double-dragon Ointment. These medicines are used for physically weak people or people suffering from a deficiency of feminine energy and internal heat.

Traditional Chinese patent medicines for invigorating the heart and strengthening the spleen: Bazhen Wan, Ginseng Yangrong Wan, Guipi Wan, Tianwang Buxin Dan and Shenqi Ointment. These medicines are used for people suffering from an insufficiency of vital energy and blood, people deficient in vital energy in their heart and spleen, and people suffering from insomnia, amnesia, mental exhaustion and physical weakness.

In the cold winter drinking a small amount of an alcoholic beverage helps to combat the cold, invigorate the blood circulation, and clear the channels of the meridian system for the flow of vital energy. Of all alcoholic beverages, wine and medicinal wines are best for middle-aged and older people, but they should not drink too much. Medicinal wine is a wine blended with traditional Chinese medicines good for increasing the vital energy and blood and strengthening muscles and bones, or a wine in which medicines are dissolved. These are good for middle-aged and older people and help improve the physique and prolong life. Medicinal wines used to cure a deficiency of vital energy in the internal organs and to cure injuries are discussed as follows.

Yanshou Jiuxian Wine: Ginseng, stir-baked Baizhu (bighead atractylodes rhizome), Fuling (Indian bread), stir-baked Gancao (licorice root), Danggui (Chinese angelica root), Chuanxiong, Shudi (prepared rehmannia root) and Baishao (white peony root), 6 g each, wolfberry 25 g, 3 large dates with pits, removed, ginger 6 g, liquor made of Chinese sorghum 1,750 ml, soaked hot for one week. Filter and remove the residue. Drink 10-15 ml at a time, once or twice a day.

Yangchun Wine: Ginseng 15 g, Baizhu (bighead atractylodes rhizome) 15 g, Shudi (prepared rehmannia root) 15 g, Danggui

(Chinese angelica root) 9 g, Tiandong (asparagus root) 9 g, Gouqizi (wolfberry) 9 g, Baiziren (arborvitae seed) 7.5 g, and Yuanzhi (milkwort root) 7.5 g. Place these into a small gauze bag, add liquor made of Chinese sorghum 2,500 ml, soak the medicines in the liquor for seven days and remove the residue from the liquid. Drink 15-20 ml at a time, once or twice a day.

Yanshou Wine: Huangjing (solomonseal rhizome) 2,000 g, Cangzhu (atractylodes rhizome) 2,000 g, Tianmendong (asparagus root) 1,500 g, pine needles 3,000 g and loquat seeds 2,500 g. Decoct these in water for 24 hours, and then make the liquor in the usual way. When ready, drink 30 ml at a time, once or twice a day.

Guben Wine: Shengdi (rehmannia root), Shudi (prepared rehmannia root), Tiandong (asparagus root), Maidong (lilyturf root), Fuling (Indian bread) and ginseng, 30 g each. Grind them into powder which is placed in a gauze bag and soaked in 1,500 ml liquor made of Chinese sorghum for three days. Then cook over low flame for 1-2 hours until the wine becomes black in color. Remove the residue and use the liquid. Drink 15-20 ml at a time, once a day.

Huangjing Wine: Huangjing (solomonseal rhizome) 200 g, Cangzhu (atractylodes rhizome) 200 g, Gouqigeng (wolfberry root) 250 g, cypress leaves 250 g, Tiandong (asparagus root) 150 g. Cook in 1,000 ml water, add distiller's yeast 500 g and glutinous rice 1,800 g to make the wine. Drink 30-50 ml at a time, twice a day.

Shuyu Wine: Shanyao (Chinese yam) 120 g, Shanyurou (dogwood fruit) 120 g, Baizhu (bighead atractylodes rhizome) 120 g, Wuweizi (magnoliavine fruit) 120 g, Fangfeng (saposhnikovia root) 90 g, ginseng 90 g, Danshen (red sage root) 90 g, and ginger 90 g. Place in a gauze bag and soak in 1,000ml rice wine for seven days. Then remove the residue from the liquid. Drink 20ml at a time, twice or three times a day.

Lurong Wine: Lurong (pilose antler) 20 g, Dongchong Xiacao (Chinese caterpillar fungus) 90 g, and liquor made of Chinese sorghum 1,500 ml. Soak for 10 days, then drink 20 ml every evening.

Tonics must be taken under the guidance of a traditional Chinese doctor. It must be first made clear whether the patient's constitution consists of the male viscera or the female viscera. People with a constitution of male viscera are not daunted by the cold, but often suffer from constipation, sore throat, toothache, dizziness, and dry and sore eyes. People with a constitution of female viscera are often strongly affected by cold in winter and may suffer from abdominal pain or loose bowels when they eat raw or cold foods. It must also be determined whether there is a deficiency of vital function or vital essence, kidney or spleen, or heart or lungs. It must also be determined whether there is a deficiency of blood in the liver or a deficiency of blood in all the organs. Only when these conditions are made clear can the doctor prescribe the proper medicines.

5. Morning, evening, day and night methods

Do climatic changes from day to night have an effect on the physiological conditions of the human body? The answer is definitely yes. The changes in nature from day and night have certain effects on the human body. Therefore, the activities of human life including work, study, physical exercise and entertainment must conform to seasonal and day-to-day changes. Once you have learned to understand the different methods of preserving health in the four seasons, it is easier to know how to preserve your health in the four different time periods of the day because the four seasons of the year correspond to the four time divisions of day, morning is equal to spring, noon to summer, evening to autumn, and night to winter. The ways to preserve health in the different periods of the day can follow the saying, "coming into being in spring, growth in summer, harvest in autumn, and hiding in winter."

The Yang *qi* (masculine energy) begins to rise in the early morning. You wake up after a night of sleep find when it dawns, you must get up. Do not get up late and do not rise too abruptly, because sudden rising is dangerous for middle-aged and old people. After you get up, you can choose an exercise according to your own interests, physical condition and surroundings. You can take a walk, run slowly, practice Taiji Quan, play Taiji Sword, practice *qigong*, play badminton or table tennis, do exercises, or ride a bicycle. When you exercise you must not overdo it. Do not exhaust yourself. Do the amount of exercise that will soothe and refresh you when you have finished.

Breakfast should be simple and light, with no greasy or hard to digest food. Generally, a porridge is the best breakfast. Because the body loses water content during a night's sleep, eating a simple and light porridge helps relax the stomach and intestines, increase the appetite, refresh the mind, improve the flow of *qi* (vital energy) and the circulation of the blood, and increase the body's immunity.

After a few hours of activity you will be hungry. You can take a rich lunch, but do not eat too quickly or overeat. It is advisable to take only 80 percent of what you want. After lunch, you may want to sleep for about an hour. Most middle-aged and older people in China like to have a nap of this length after lunch. You will awake refreshed, vigorous, and ready to work efficiently. This is a good habit and should be encouraged.

For supper, you should eat easily digested and nutritious food. Do not go to bed right after supper, but instead take a walk outdoor and stretch yourself, with little physical exertion. Do not over-stress your bones and muscles in the evening or sleep too late. An old saying goes: "It's good for health if you go to sleep and rise early."

Be sure to get eight hours of sleep. Eating and sleeping well are two essential requirements for keeping physically fit. They are also the signs of good health, most healthy old people are in tune with these two conditions.

To sum up, if a person can be accomodated to changes in the natural surroundings, and take proper measures to preserve health in conformity climatic changes during the year and during each day, he will be free from illness and enjoy good health and a long life.

Chapter Two

Methods of Purging One's Mind of Ambitions and Desires

What does "purging one's mind of ambitions and desires" mean? It means that one should strive for a peaceful state of mind, one without ambitions and desires. We will deal with this question in six aspects.

1. Cultivate moral character

Character cultivation and being even-tempered have direct bearing on health and longeveity. Generally if a man has cultivated his moral character well, he will have a longer life, and if he has cultivated his moral character not so well, a shorter life may be his fate. Therefore, a man should do good deeds and be happy to help others, especially those in need, and regard the needs of others as his own. If he does this, it shows a broad mind, one not preoccupied with personal gain. When he helps others, he is happy and this is good for his health. And once you help others, they will also help you. When you are in need, those who once received your aid will lend their hand and help you out of difficulty.

There is an old saying in China: "Performing a charitable deed can cure illness, and doing a pious deed can help prolong life." A man who is kind and honest and does no harm to others has a good temper, smooth circulation of *qi* (vital energy) and blood, strong immunity, and good nervous and internal systems, and he seldom falls ill. A man who harbors ill intentions and harms others to benefit himself often suffers nervous system and internal disorders, and therefore develops weak immunity causing disease and even early death.

The great pharmacologist Sun Simiao lived over 100 years. He was still strong and vigorous even in old age. His book *Qian Jin Yao Fang* (*The Thousand Golden Formulae*) has been used as an encyclopedia of clinical medicine for generations. In the chapter of "Character Cultivation" of the book he wrote: "Those who cultivate their moral character by doing charitable deeds never fall seriously ill or suffer calamities. This is the great principle for keeping good health." Character cultivation means moral character cultivation. It is a long process. After years of cultivation and tempering you get into the habit, and your temper becomes naturally good.

Apart from moral character cultivation, it is also very important to remold and temper character. A person who has a narrow mind and a short temper is introverted and often feel depressed. Such a one was Lin Daiyu in the classic Chinese novel *A Dream of Red Mansions*. She could hardly stand to hear one word from others, and often shed tears over small trifles. Tears accompanied her every day of her life, so she was weak and frequently ill, and died before she was 20. It is a pity and a sorrow that a beautiful and talented girl like her did not have time to enjoy whatever a girl deserves after she comes into the world.

2. Do not be greedy

It is well said: "People walk toward the high, while water flows toward the low." It is the human nature to eagerly seek the upper hand and strive to do well in everything. This is not a bad thing. Only when one is eager to get the upper hand and to do well does one have the desire to do better and the motivation to make progress. However, if he is blindly bent on seeking fame and high position and scrambles for them by force and trickery without considering his objective conditions and surroundings, he will be upset, dejected and unhappy when his goals are not realized. Some fall ill, some die early, and some even commit suicide, and some are killed in the scramble.

Whether seeking fame, money or high position, one should try to achieve them on the basis of their ability and objective conditions, but never overdo it or be too greedy for them. A saying goes: "One is always happy to feel content with his lot." Only when he "is content with his lot," can he be "always happy." Only when he is "not greedy," can he be "content with his lot." Only when he has "a peaceful state of mind and has no desires," can he be "not greedy." Therefore, if you want to be healthy and enjoy a long life, "having a peaceful mind and no desires" is the foundation.

If you have no wild desires, you will find it very easy to be content. In this way you maintain a calm mind, good health, and may look forward to a long life.

Lao Zi says: "No disaster is greater than not being content, and no blame is larger than the desire for gain. Therefore, it is good to feel content with your lot, and stop at that."

3. Free oneself of worries

There are many ways to dispel sadness, grief and worry, and people can choose the one best suited to their own circumstances. The following are only for your reference:

Give vent to your vexation. If you do not, and hide it in your heart for a long time, this can be disastrous to you health. When you are upset you should tell your family or your best friends about it and listen to their advice. Or write all your grievances, injustice, grief, and worry in a diary. You may even cry aloud to vent your grief, or you can run or shout wildly in the outskirts to give vent to it.

Change your temperament and interests. When one thing troubles you, you can shift your attention to other things. Do not linger on thought of unsatisfactory things. You can play chess, play cards, go to theater, fly a kite, relax yourself. Or you can travel to a scenic spot and visit ancient temples, using the beautiful scenery to mold your temperament, shift your interest, and broaden your mind.

Be open-minded, magnanimous and optimistic. When you are dissatisfied, you should realize that others may be as well. When you continue to worry, you will find yourself even more bogged down in your grievances and become even more narrow-minded. The narrow-mindedness causes you to indulge yourself in blind worry. If you analyze the situation and exercise forbearance, your mind will become broad, your mood optimistic, and your worries and depression will be easily dispelled.

4. Harmonious family

A harmonious family is very important to the middle-aged and older people. The family not only provides a place to live, but also a "realm of freedom." In your family, you can enjoy freedom, love and warmth to your heart's content. Generally, all people in good health and who enjoy longevity have a warm and harmonious family. When you are worried, your family comforts you. When you are tired or sick, your family takes care of you. When you achieve, your family shares your happiness. And when you are in need, the family meets together to share your difficulty. A perfect and happy family makes every member happy. Not only do you work with full energy, but the family helps you to achieve success in your career. It is also beneficial to your health. On the contrary, if couple falls out, or their children are not good to them, the family becomes like an ice cave where there is no warmth. The family members are cold to each other and show no warm feelings. When you come home after a day's work, you feel even more depressed. If you are unsuccessful in your work, you get no consoling words, but only cold eyes, grievances and ridicules. When you fall sick and must recuperate at home, you get no care but only ironical words, or even maltreatment. Such a family inevitably does harm to your health and may lead to an early decline. Therefore, to keep in good health, an harmonious family is absolutely essential.

How does one maintain an harmonious family? First comes mutual love between the husband and wife. The couple is the mainstay of the family, and good and harmonious relations between them guarantees harmonious relations among all family members. The husband and wife should respect and love each other and manage family affairs together.

Secondly, they show respect for elders and love for the young. The elders have worked their whole life, and they should be taken care of and supported so they can be happy in their later years. Your parents are your first teachers. If you show them respect and piety, your children will do the same when you are old. If you do not, neither will your children. The family style is traditional, passed down from generation to generation.

The children are the future and hope of the nation. Care should be taken so they grow up healthily. They should be educated to show respect for their parents and grandparents, as well as their teachers and all older people.

An old saying goes: "It's better to have a good daughter-in-law than to have a good son, and it's better to have a good son-in-law than to have a good daughter." The husband should show love and respect for his parents-in-law and the wife should do the same. Only in this way can family relations go well and the love between husband and wife be further deepened for a more harmonious family. If you are a stepfather or stepmother, you should show special love for your stepchildren. Only in this way can family relations become more harmonious. If you maltreat the children of others, you will not only receive condemnation from society, but fall out with your new spouse.

5. Interpersonal relations

Apart from family relations, relations with other people are also very important. These include relations with your colleagues, friends and relatives. If all these relations are well handled, it will also benefit your health. If you have good relations with everyone, you will get help from your friends and get along smoothly at work. In this way, you naturally have an easy mind, feel content and happy, and enjoy good health. This helps to delay the aging process.

There are many ways of maintaining good relations with other people. The main way is to show respect for others. When you respect others, you will be respected. It is mutual. Moreover, you should be sincere and honest if you want to be trusted. Third, you should be glad to help others. When you do this, they will also help you in time of need.

Chapter Three

Eating and Drinking Moderately*

1. Eat and drink moderately

Building health by eating the right food is closely related to long life. In traditional Chinese ways to preserve health, nutritious food is of paramount importance. From ancient times China has accumulated a rich experience in this regard.

Eating and drinking in moderation means eating neither too little nor too much. If you eat too little, the nutrition will be insufficient to meet the needs of your body, and you may suffer from malnutrition or "deficiency of vital energy and lowering of body resistance" as it is called in the traditional Chinese medicine. If you eat too much once in a while, this may hurt your spleen and stomach, and you may suffer from nausea, vomiting, and bone ache. Especially if you eat too much in the evening you will find it hard to digest and this will affect your sleep. This is what traditional Chinese medicine calls "if the stomach is not soothing, the sleep will be disturbed."

If you eat too much fish, chicken, meat and eggs with high fat content for a long time, this can easily cause the accumulation of internal heat and ulcers. If you have a good appetite and eat out of control, you will suffer from obesity, diabetes, hypertension and coronary heart disease, thus accelerating aging process. Referring

---

*Chinese food, tea, and traditional Chinese medicines, prepared by pharmacies described in this chapter are available in Chinatowns throughout the world.

to the harm done by overeating, an ancient Chinese physician said: "Those who eat too much have five disadvantages: 1. excess of stool (loose bowels caused by the harm done to the intestines and stomach), 2. excess of urine (diabetes caused by excessive fat), 3. disturbance of sleep, 4. overweight with ugly body form, and 5. indigestion."

2. Quality of food and drink

To ensure good health and the body's needs, it is essential to take all kinds of nutriments. So food and drink should be diversified. There should be both meat dishes and vegetarian dishes, both vegetables and fruits. A reasonable combination of meats and vegetables can ensure the body's needs. Some of the nutriments in meat are not available in vegetarian food. So you must not go on a vegetarian diet. Giving up meat and fish is harmful to health. Even a vegetarian diet must be all-inclusive, not monotonous.

From long practice, people have come to realize that a greedy appetite for greasy and rich foods is liable to cause ulcers and diabetes. Modern medical research has shown that if too much fat is absorbed, the fat is deposited in the body and attaches to the walls of the blood vessels, causing arteriosclerosis. It may also cause fatty heart and liver. If deposited beneath the skin or in the abdominal cavity, it causes obesity. Meats, especially internal organs, have a high cholesterol content. Too much cholesterol contained in the blood and deposited on the walls of the arteries will lead to arteriosclerosis and hypertension, coronary heart disease and cerebral apoplexy. The inference made by traditional Chinese medicine that middle-aged and old people should eat more vegetarian food turns out to be a scientific one.

Middle-aged and old people should eat foods with less fats. It is good for them to eat bean oil, sunflower-seed oil, rape oil and cheese.

Besides vegetarian food, the ancient Chinese physicians also advocated light and simple food. Light and simple food does not mean bland food, but rather that the five flavors — sour, bitter, sweet, pungent and salty — must not be too heavy. The 2,000-year-old Chinese medical classic *The Yellow Emperor's Canon of Medicine* warned in the volume *Questions and Answers*: "If you eat too much salty food, your blood vessels thicken and become dark in color; if you eat too much bitter food, your skin becomes dry and you lose your hair; if you eat too much pungent food, your sinews become tight and your nails become dry; if you eat too much sour food, your skin and flesh become thick and shrink and your lips become dry and chap; and if you eat too much sweet food, it will harm the bones, and you will lose your hair." Among the five flavors, salt in particular should be used moderately. Ancient Chinese physicians warned against eating too much salt, and modern medical research has demonstrated that many diseases including hypertension, coronary heart disease, arteriosclerosis, cirrhosis of the liver, cerebral apoplexy, kidney diseases, and cancer of the esophagus are related to eating too much salt.

3. Balance of the three meals

Adults usually eat three meals a day and the intervals between them are usually around five hours. This conforms to normal physiological conditions because food usually remains in the stomach for 4-5 hours. If the interval between meals is too long, you become hungry, if too short, the digestive system does not have time to function and this affects the appetite and digestion. Studies confirm that if one eats three meals a day, the intestines and stomach can fully absorb all the nutriments in the food. Of what then should the three meals consist? A Chinese saying goes: "Eat well for breakfast, eat full at lunch, and eat less for supper." By eating well and full for the breakfast and lunch, you can absorb the nutriments fully and guarantee the energy needed for a day's work or physical activities. Otherwise, you may suffer from blood sugar deficiency, palpitations, dizziness, absent-mindedness or fatigue. If you eat too much for supper and sleep on a full stomach, you may suffer from indigestion, obesity, hypertension or coronary heart disease. For coronary heart disease sufferers in particular, there is the danger of an abrupt occurrence of myocardial infarction during sleep if they eat too much greasy and sweet food before sleep. Middle-aged and older people should be aware of this.

4. Taste in food

Everyone has his own taste in food and drink. Some like sweet food, others like sour food, some like hot foods, some like salty food, some like meat and greasy food, and so on. However, if one likes to eat a particular food too much and fails to control it consciously, this inevitably causes too much of certain nutriments to be deposited in the body, while others remain insufficient. This leads to partial growth and partial decline of Yin and Yang and may cause disease. For example, rickets is caused by a deficiency of calcium, and calcium is found abundant in vegetables, fruits, beans, milk, eggs, and other food. You can eat these foods to prevent and cure rickets. Night blindness is caused by a deficiency of vitamins A and D, and they are plentiful in the fish and livers. Scurvy is caused by a deficiency of vitamin C, and vitamin C is available in fresh fruits and vegetables. Beriberi is caused by a deficiency of vitamin B, and vitamin B is found in coarse rice and wheat flour.

Then can we eat too much? The answer is no. If you eat any

food too much it may cause illness. If you eat too much fruit and melon, it may harm your intestines and stomach, causing loose bowels, vomiting and stomachache. If you eat too much food with high fat and caloric content, it may lead to damp-heat in the body, turbidity and clogging of phlegm, bleeding piles, and boils. If you eat too much sour food it may lead to a luxuriant growth of liver energy, the weakening of spleen energy, and cause abdominal distention and hypochondria. If you eat too much sweet foods, this may cause blackening facial color and irritability in the chest. If you eat too much bitter food it may harm the spleen and stomach, causing indigestion and a bloated stomach. If you eat too much pungent food, the sinews and veins may become flaccid. And, finally, if you eat too much salty food, this may harm the muscles and bones, causing amyotrophy and depression.

One must eat all kinds of foods, both coarse grains and fine grains, meat and vegetarian dishes, and vegetables and fruits. Only in this may can you ensure the supply of all nutriments and promote health and long life.

5. Alcoholic beverages, tea, and health preservation

Traditional Chinese medicine holds that alcoholic beverages help clear the channels of the meridian system for the smooth flow of vital energy, the circulation of *qi* and blood, and the regulation of blood flow to distribute strength to all parts of the body. Drinking small amounts of alcoholic beverages can therefore be beneficial to health. Modern research has shown that good-quality liquor contains more than 70 aromatic elements, many of which are essential to health. Wine also contains rich nutrients which help strengthen the stomach and other parts of the body. Rice wine has an even greater nutritional value since it contains dextrin, carbohydrate, organic acids, multiple vitamins, and 17 amino acids, seven of which are essential but cannot be synthesized in the body. Medicinal liquor has a great tonic effect. Alcoholic beverages also promote the secretion of UK urokinase, an enzyme which is the best substance for dissolving blood clots. Therefore, drinking a small amount of alcoholic beverages can help prevent myocardial infarction and cerebral thrombus.

However, drinking alcohol must be done in moderation. One must not become addicted to alcohol. Extensive drinking over a long time does harm to the cerebral tissue and causes cerebral atrophy. It also harms the reproductive cells, causing lowered intelligence or congenital malformation in children. It can also damage the liver cells, causing cirrhosis. Extended alcoholic drinks can also result in magnesium, iron, copper, protein, and multiple vitamin, deficiency giving rise to undernourishment and low immunity. What is a moderate amount of wine drinking? This depends on the person and the type of alcoholic beverage. Generally, with hard liquor, 20-30 ml at a time is enough, certainly no more than 50 ml at most. For rice wine or grape wine, 30-50 ml a day is fine. For the methods of compounding medicinal wines and the proper amount of wine, please refer to the preceding chapter "Seasonal Methods : Winter" or see a doctor for advice. For some people it is best not to drink alcoholic beverages at all. These include patients with hot diseases, inflammation, and those taking furazolidone, aspirin, nitroglycerine, phenytoin sodium, metronidazole, drugs for reducing blood sugar, and anti-allergic drugs. Moreover, who often suffer from dry bowels, toothache, sore throat and headache or people allergic to alcohol are also advised not to drink alcoholic beverages.

China is the home of tea, with a tea-drinking history of more than 5,000 years. The Chinese forefathers long ago knew the medicinal value of tea for preserving health. Its earliest book on herbal medicine *Shen Nong's Materia Medica* says: "Tea tastes bitter.

When you drink it, it benefits your brain, makes you less sleepy and refreshed and improves your sight." In the Ming Dynasty, Li Shizhen wrote of the medicinal value of tea in his book *Compendium of Materia Medica*: "Tea is bitter and sweet, slightly cold, but poisonless. It cures haemorrhoids, fistula, and heart thirst. It is diuretic, dispels phlegm-heat, checks the upward flow of vital energy, and improves the digestion."

Over thousands of years the Chinese people have accumulated a very rich experience in the use of medicinal tea to preserve health. In the following, we would like to introduce some of these teas:

Black tea: The fresh tea leaves are kneaded or rubbed, fermented and dried. Chinese black tea reduces blood lipids thereby softening the blood vessels, promoting blood circulation to remove blood stasis, and clearing the cerebrum of internal fire to refresh the mind.

Green tea: Fresh tea leaves are rubbed and dried without fermenting. The varieties of Chinese green teas are Tun, Wu, Hang, and Xiang. The Longjing green tea grown in Hangzhou and the Maojian green tea grown in Xinyang are both famous green teas. Chinese green tea promotes blood circulation in the brain to refresh the mind, clears away internal heat to facilitate the excretion of urine, and eliminates inflammation to relieve internal heat.

Jasmine tea: This is a black tea blended with jasmine flowers, fragrant and refreshing.

Milk tea and butter tea: Cook the tea with cow milk, sheep milk or butter. Apart from having the same effect as black tea and green tea, it has a very high nutritional value and is good for middle-aged and old people and the physically weak. This tea is very popular among people of the ethnic nationalities in the livestock-breeding regions of Tibet, Xinjiang, Qinghai, Ningxia and Inner Mongolia.

Honeysuckle tea: Put 3 g honeysuckle and 1 g tea together and pour in hot water. This tea helps clear away internal heat to remove toxic substance and cure ulcers and the flu.

Peppermint tea: Put 2 g dried peppermint leaves (or 6 g fresh leaves) and 1 g tea, and pour in boiling water. This will help cure flu, headache, toothache, and acute nasosinusitis.

Black plum tea: Take 3 fresh black plums and crush them, then mix them with 1 g tea, and 6 g white sugar or iced sugar. Pour in boiling water. This promotes the secretion of saliva to relieve thirst, clearing away heat and increasing the appetite.

Bamboo leaf tea: Take 3 g dried bamboo leaves (or 6 g fresh leaves), and 1 g tea, pour in boiling water. This clears the heart heat to eliminate irritation, clears away heat to promote the excretion of urine, and helps cure mental irritability and bacterial infection of the urinary organs.

Sorghum stem skin tea: Strip the skin of the sorghum stem, burn it over a charcoal fire until it becomes brown, and cut into small pieces. Use 3 g each time with 1 g tea, and pour in boiling water. This helps cure inflammation of the urinary tract and bladder, and bacterial infection in all urinary organs.

Chrysanthemum tea: Take 3 g chrysanthemum flowers and 1 g tea, pour in boiling water. This tea clears liver of heat to improve sight, and helps cure dizziness, headache and hypertension.

Haw tea: Take 10 g dried haws (or 30 g fresh ones), crush them, add 200 ml water and boil them for 20 minutes. Turn off the flame and add 1.5 g tea leaves. Filter the liquid when it cools and drink. This tea helps improve the digestion, kills germs, removes blood stasis, and reduces blood lipids. This tea is used to treat indigestion, postpartum abdominal pains and incessant postpartum lochia, bacterial dysentery, high blood lipids, and obesity.

Mung bean tea: Take 30 g mung beans and 300 ml water. Boil them for 40 minutes and then turn off the flame. Add 1.5 g tea leaves. Drink slowly after it cools. This tea clears away heat, detoxifying and relieving the summer heat and swelling. It also helps cure heatstroke, irritability and thirst, dizziness, headache, toothache, and sore throat.

Turnip tea: Take 60 g fresh turnip (or 30 g dried turnip) and 500 ml water. Boil them for 1 hour. Add 5 g tea leaves after turning off the flame. Remove the residue after five minutes and drink. This helps relieve carbon monoxide poisoning.

Chuanxiong tea: Take 6 g chuanxiong (dried rhizome of Ligusticum chuanxiong) and 250 ml water. Boil them for 10 minutes before adding 3 g tea leaves. Immediately turn off flame. Drink after it cools. This tea helps to cure headache, dysmenorrhoea and delayed menstruation.

Perilla leaf tea: Take 15 g perilla leaves (30 g fresh perilla leaves) and 500 ml water. Boil the perilla for 15 minutes. Add 1.5 g tea leaves after turning off the flame and stopping the fire, and drink when it becomes lukewarm. This tea is good for relieving poisoning caused by eating crabs and fish.

Giant-hyssop tea: Take 15 g giant-hyssop leaves (30g fresh leaves) and 300 ml water. Boil them for 10 minutes and add 2 g black tea after turning off the flame. Drink when lukewarm. This tea is used to cure stomachache, loose bowels, nausea, vomiting, headache and dizziness caused by over exposure to cold air and consuming cold drinks in summer.

Modern research has discovered that tea contains vitamins C and B which are used to treat leprosy, scurvy, beriberi, inflammation of the mouth corners, dry skin cracks, scalp favus, alopecia areata, acne, and menstrual disorders. Tea also contains tannic acid which has an astringent effect. Theine is good for refreshing the mind, dilating the blood vessels, facilitating the excretion of urine, and lowering blood pressure. Theophylline helps dilate the blood vessels and break up colesterol. Tea pigments help prevent and treat arteriosclerosis. Longtime tea-drinking may help prevent cancer, prevent and treat coronary heart disease, pulmonary heart disease and bronchitis, and at the same time improve the function of the central nervous system, strengthen metabolism, increase beauty, and prolong life. Investigations show that of the 11 people over the age of 100 in Chengdu, in southwest China, nine are longtime tea drinkers.

Tea drinking benefits the human body, but attention should be paid to the scientific way of drinking. For example, you should refrain from drinking too much strong tea before bedtime, as tea is a stimulant and may cause insomnia. Tea is also a diuretic. If you drink too much it will increase urination at night and disturb your sleep. It also is not advisable to drink tea after meals because the tannin in the tea combines quickly with protein and other nutrients to form sediments which harm digestion and absorption. Do not use tea when taking medicine because the tannic substance also easily combines with the medicine to change its properties and reduce effectiveness. Do not pour boiling water on tea, because the high temperature of the boiling water destroys the vitamin C in the tea and volatilizes its fragrance.

6. Nutritional food

As the constitution of middle-aged and old people begin to decline, they need the replenishment of various nutrients. If they are deficient in this or that nutriment, they may begin to decline early, thus affecting their chances for a long life.

Chinese doctors have always attached great importance to the efficacy of food. Zhang Congzheng, a physician of the Jin Dynasty (1115-1234), said that health building depends on eating nourishing food, while curing illness depends on taking medicines. The blending of different nutrients has been described in the first three sections of this chapter. Then how can middle-aged and old people know the proper foods to eat?

Spring: In spring the Yang *qi* (masculine energy) rises. Then it is best to eat food with a warm nature, as this promotes the rise of masculine energy. Barley, wheat, large dates and peanuts support Yang *qi*. It is not good to eat glutinous, greasy or cold food, as this harms the spleen and stomach and affects digestion.

Summer: It is hot in summer, both *qi* (vital energy) and the blood flow to the surface of the body with Yang *qi* coming out and Yin *qi* staying inside. In this season, it is better to eat foods that help to clear away the summer heat, reinforce vital energy, and promote the secretion of saliva. Such foods are mung bean soup, hyacinth bean soup, sweet-sour plum juice, round-grained non-glutinous rice porridge, lotus leaf rice porridge, watermelon and strawberries. It is also advisable to drink green tea, bamboo leaf tea, and honeysuckle flower tea (please refer to the section "Alcoholic beverages, Tea and Health Preservation" in this chapter for details).

Autumn: Hu Sihui, a health specialist of the Yuan Dynasty (1206-1368), said: "It is dry in autumn, then it is good to eat sesame to moisten the dryness." In addition, it is also good to eat round-grained non-glutinous rice, glutinous rice, honey, milk, pineapple, loquats, water chestnuts, Chinese yam, sugar cane, and pears. It is also advisable not to eat too much hot pepper, onion, or garlic.

Winter: During the cold season more calories are consumed. From ancient times Chinese people have known about eating nourishing food in winter. Most nourishing foods have warm properties. In traditional Chinese medical theory, Chinese medicines are divided into four categories according to their respective properties: cold, hot, warm and cool. Cold and cool medicines help reduce internal heat, while warm and hot medicines help warm the spleen and stomach to dispel cold. Likewise, traditional Chinese medicine also divides food into four categories: cold, hot, warm and cool. Foods with warm and hot properties are good in winter, while foods with cold and cool properties are good in summer. Foods with warm and hot properties include broomcorn millet, millet, large dates, walnut kernels, lotus seeds, fungus, fish, beef and mutton. These are all nutritious foods for winter.

7. Nourishment through medicines

The nutritional value of Chinese medicines was recognized long ago, and they continue to be widely used in medical practice for maintaining health and prolonging life.

As early as 1,800 years ago, Hua Tuo, a famous physician during the latter years of the Eastern Han Dynasty(25-220), gave his medical prescription for protecting health and prolonging life called "qiyeqingzhansan" powder to his disciple named Fan Ah. Fan Ah persisted in taking the powder and lived over 100 years. This powder is a Chinese medicine called solomonseal rhizome. It has the effect of greatly nourishing the semen, vital energy and blood. Modern medical research has found that solomonseal rhizome increases the T lymphocytes in the human body and helps reduce blood sugar and cholesterol, thus helping prevent and cure cardiovascular diseases and diabetes.

Li Shizhen, a great Ming Dynasty physician recorded a story of eating wolfberry to prolong life in his *Compendium of Materia Medica*. Through many investigations, he came to the conclusion that wolfberry was sweet, mild and poisonless, "strengthens the muscles and bones, keeps one vigorous and young, ...improves the eyesight, eases mental strain, and prolongs life if one keeps taking it for a long time." Modern medical research has found that wolfberry does indeed reduce blood pressure and blood sugar, dilate the blood vessels, increase the T lymphocytes and improve the body's immunity function. It also helps cure the fatty liver, hypertension, coronary heart disease, diabetes and arteriosclerosis, and helps resist aging and senile decline to prolong life.

Chinese medicine for nourishing the blood includes Danggui (Chinese angelica root), Shudi (prepared rehmannia root), Baishao (white peony root), Danshen (red sage root), Heshouwu (fleeceflower root), Ejiao (ass-hide glue), Longyanrou (longan aril), Huangjing (solomonseal rhizome), mulberry fruit, wolfberry and Jixueteng (spatholobus stem).

Chinese medicine for replenishing vital energy includes ginseng, Dangshen (Asiabell root), Huangqi (milkvetch root), Baizhu (bighead atractylodes rhizome), Shanyao (Chinese yam), Baibiandou (white hyacinth bean), Gancao (licorice root), Chinese date, malt extract and bee honey.

Chinese medicine for nourishing Yin *qi* includes Shashen (straight ladybell root), Maidong (lilyturf root), Shihu (dendrobium), Yuzhu (fragrant solomonseal rhizome), Baihe (lily), Nuzhenzi (grossy privet fruit), and Shengdihuang (rehmannia root).

Chinese medcine for invigorating Yang *qi* includes Lurong (pilose antler), Roucongrong (cistanche), Duzhong (eucommia bark), Xuduan (teasel root), Gouji (cibot rhizome), Gusuibu (drynaria rhizome), Yizhiren (sharpleaf galangal seed), Dongchongxiacao (Chinese caterpillar fungus), Gejie (gecko), walnut kernel, Ziheche (human placenta), Tusizi (dodder seed), Shayuanzi (flatstem milkvetch seed), Suoyang (cynomorium), Jiuzi (chive seeds), and Yangqishi (actinolite).

Following are some secret recipes for long life for your reference: Yanling Yishou Pellets (Selected Prescriptions for Empress

Dowager Cixi and Emperor Guangxu of the Qing Dynasty with Remarks)

Ingredients: Fushen, Fuling (Indian bread) and Danggui (Chinese angelica root), 18g each, Hangbaishao (white peony root from Hangzhou), Yebaizhu (wild bighead atractylodes), Chaodangshen (stir-baked Asiabell root), Jiuhuangqi (stir-baked milkvetch root with adjuvant), dried tangerine peel, Xiangfu (flatsedge tuber), and stir-baked date pit kernel, 12 g each, Yuanzhi (milkwort root), Guangmuxiang (costus root), Sharen (spiny amomum fruit), Shichangpu (grass-leaved sweetflag rhizome) and longan, 9 g each, Jiugancao (stir-baked licorice root) with adjuvant 6 g.

Methods of preparation and administration: Pestle these ingredients into powder, make pellets with honey as big as a mung bean, use cinnabar for its coating. Take 6 g at a time with boiled water, two or three times a day. It has the effect of reinforcing vital energy and blood, nourishing the heart and spleen, relieving the mental strain and maintaining tranquility, and helps to cure anxiety, deficiency of vital energy and blood, poor appetite and physical weakness, constipation, insomnia and amnesia.

Changchun Yishou Pellets (Selected Prescriptions for Empress Dowager Cixi and Emperor Guangxu of the Qing Dynasty with Remarks)

Ingredients: Tianmendong (asparagus root, with the heart removed), Maidong (lilyturf root, with the heart removed), Shudi (prepared rehmannia root), Shanyao (Chinese yam), Niuxi (two-toothed achyranthes root), Shengdihuang (rehmannia root), Chaoduzhong (stir-baked eucommia bark), Shanzhuyu (dogwood fruit), Baifuling (white Indian bread), ginseng, Wuweizi (magnoliavine fruit), Muxiang (costus root), Bajitian (morinda root), and Baiziren (arborvitae seed kernel), 60 g each, Chuanjiao (chuanjiao, slightly stir-baked, leaving out those with eyes and closed mouth), Zixie (water-plantain tuber), Shichangpu (grass-leaved sweetflag rhizome), Yuanzhi (milkwort root), 30 g each, Tusizi (dodder seed) and Roucongrong (cistanche), 120 g each, wolfberry, wolfberry bark and raspberry, 45 g each.

Methods of preparation and administration: Pestle the ingredients into powder, make pellets with honey as big as the Chinese parasol seed. Take 50 pellets at a time in the beginning, 60 pellets after 30 days, and 80 pellets after 100 days, once every morning with lightly salted water. It has the effect in nourishing the liver, strengthening the waist and knees, invigorating the semen and blood, and improving mental ability, and helps to cure the early whitening of beard and hair, declining energy and weak and sore back and knees.

Yangxin Yannian Yishou Pellets (Selected Prescriptions for Empress Dowager Cixi and Guangxu of the Qing Dynasty with Remarks)

Ingredients: Fushen, Jiuchao Danggui (Chinese angelica root stir-baked with wine), Danshen (red sage root), Baiziren (arborvitae seed kernel), Jiubaishao (wine-treated white peony root), Mudanpi (tree peony bark), Gandihuang (dried rehmannia root), Chaozhiqiao (stir-baked bitter orange), and Suanzaoren (spiny jujube pit kernel), 18g each, Chuanxiong, Chaobaizhu (stir-baked bighead atractylodes), tangerine peel, Jiuhuangling (wine- treated skullcap root), and Zhizi (cape-jasmine fruit), 10 g each.

Methods of preparation and administration: Pestle the ingredients into powder, make pellets with honey as big as a mung bean, and use cinnabar for its coating. Take 6 g at a time with boiled water, twice or three times a day. It has the effect of nourishing the heart to maintain tranquility, clearing the liver of internal heat, invigorating the spleen, and prolonging life. It also helps cure excessive liver fire, deficiency of both heart and spleen, insufficiency of vital energy, insomnia due to deficiency of Yin, dry throat, and heat in the palm and sole.

Baoyuan Yishou Pellets (Selected Prescriptions for Empress Dowager Cixi and Emperor Guangxu of the Qing Dynasty with Remarks)

Ingredients: Ginseng and Baizhu (bighead atractylodes), 10 g each, Gandihuang (dried rehmannia root), Danggui (Chinese angelica root), Chaoduzhong (stir-baked eucommia bark), Chaoguya (stir-baked germinated millet), and mulberry twig, 15 g each, Chaoyimi (stir-baked job's tear seeds) and Fuling (Indian bread), 18 g each, Chaobaishao (stir-baked white peony root), Jiuxiangfu (stir-baked flatsedge tuber with adjuvant) and balloonflower, 6 g each, tangerine peel, Sharen (spiny amomum fruit), Cuzihu (vinegar-treated Chinese thoroughwax root), and Jiugancao (stir-baked licorice root with adjuvant), 3 g each.

Methods of preparation and administration: Pestle the ingredients into powder. Take 4 g with millet soup at a time, twice a day. It has the effect of replenishing vital energy and blood, and regulating the functions of the liver and spleen. It helps to cure the disharmony of the liver and spleen, deficiency of both vital energy and blood, dizziness and mental fatigue, lack of appetite, and watery stool.

These four prescriptions were frequently used by the Empress Dowager Cixi of the Qing Dynasty. By taking these drugs she lived 73 years, much longer than the average life-span of 50 years at that time.

Shouwu Yanshou Pellets (*Shi Bu Zhai Medical Book*)

Ingredients: Heshouwu (fleeceflower root) 300 g, Xixiancao (common St. Paulswort), mulberry fruit extract, black sesame seeds extract, Jinyingzi (cherokee rose-hip) extract, Hanliancao (eclipta prostrata) extract and Tusizi (dodder seed), 60 g each, Chaoduzhong (stir-baked eucommia bark), Niuxi (two-toothed achyranthes), Nuzhenzi (grossy privet fruit) and Shuangsangye (red mulberry leaves), 30 g each, Rendongteng (honeysuckle vine) and Shengdi (rehmannia root), 15 g each.

Methods of preparation and administration: Pestle the ingredients (except for the extracts) into powder, add the extracts and mix them with heated white honey to make pellets the size of a Chinese parasol seed. Take 4 g with boiled water, three times a day. It has the effect of prolonging life.

This prescription was passed down by Dong Qichang (1555-1636), a famous calligrapher and painter of the Ming Dynasty. After he took the pellets in his old age, his white hair returned to black and he became very energetic and lived 81 years. The high officials and noble lords of the Qing Dynasty took the pellets to keep in good health and prolonging their life. Liang Zhangju, a man of letters, and Lu Maoxiu, a physician, both of the Qing Dynasty, spoke highly of this prescription.

Qianjin Bulao Pellets (*Qian Jin Yi Fang* [*Supplement to the Thousand Golden Formulae*])

Ingredients: Shengshanyao (Chinese yam) 60 g, Roucongrong (cistanche) 120 g, Wuweizi (magnoliavine fruit) 100 g, Tusizi (dodder seed) and Chaoduzhong (stir-baked eucommia bark), 90 g each, Niuxi (two-toothed achyranthes root), Zexie (water-plantain tuber), Shengdi (rehmannia root), Shanzhuyu (dogwood fruit), Fu-shen, Bajitian (morinda root) and Chishizhi (red halloysite), 30 g each.

Methods of preparation and administration: Pestle the ingredients into powder, make pellets with honey the size of a Chinese parasol seed. Take 15 pellets with warm rice wine before meals, twice a day, every morning and evening. Avoid vinegar, garlic and fermented foods with foul odor. This prescription was handed down by Sun Simiao, a great physician of the Tang Dynasty (618-907). By taking the pellets, he lived 101 years (581-682). In recent years, people have tested this prescription handed down from ancient times and have found that it improves health and prolongs life. Generally, old people have a sleek face, rosy lips, warm limbs and full vigor after taking these pellets for one week.

Yansheng Hubao Pellets (*Prescriptions of the Imperial Hospital*)

Ingredients: Tusizi (dodder seed, washed clean in water, soaked in wine and baked dry to use as powder) and Chinese dates (pits removed and baked dry), 90 g each, Jiucaizi (chive seeds, washed clean in water, soaked in wine for 12 hours, and baked dry over low fire) 120 g, Roucongrong (cistanche, cut into slices after it is soaked in wine, and baked dry), Shechuangzi (cnidium fruit, washed clean in water and baked dry) and Wancan'e (late silk moth, stir-fried in butter over low fire), 60 g each, Shenglonggu (dragon's bone, wrapped in cloth and soaked in well water for 12 hours), Lurong (pilose antler with the hair removed), Sangpiaoxiao (mantis egg-case, stir-baked), lotus seeds (skin removed and stir-baked until done), dried lotus flower stamen, Huluba (fenugreek seed, slightly stir-baked), 30 g each, Muxiang (costus root), Dingxiang (cloves) and Nanruxiang (frankincense), 15 g each, and musk 6 g.

Methods of preparation and administration: Pestle the ingredients separately into powder. First put 6 kilograms of wine together with the Tusizi (dodder seed) powder, and decoct it over a low fire until half remains, add 30 g buckwheat flour and mix well, then put in the other 14 ingredients in order, the last being musk. Keep stirring when the ingredients are put in one by one until the decoction becomes an ointment. If the decoction is already too thick before all ingredients are put in, add more wine at any time to avoid the hardening of the ointment. After the extract is ready, make it into pellets each the size of a Chinese parasol seed. Take 15 pellets with warm wine or lightly salted water every morning before breakfast. Sit calmly for 5-6 minutes after taking the pellets. If the masculine energy (Yang *qi*) is declining too much, take it for a second time in the evening. This prescription is said to improve the kidneys to invigorate Yang or masculine energy, and help cure impotence and involuntary emission, sore waist and knees, increased urination at night, exhaustion and listlessness, and sexual malfunction.

Wuxu Jianyang Pellets (*Wan's Jishan Hall Proven Secret Recipes for Nourishment*)

Ingredients: Chishouwu (red fleeceflower root), Baishouwu (white fleeceflower root), Chifuling (red Indian bread) and Baifuling (white Indian bread), 500 g each, Niuxi (two-toothed achyranthes), Danggui (Chinese angelica root), Qiguo (wolfberry fruit) and Tusizi (dodder seed), 240 g each, and Buguzhi (scurfpea fruit) 120 g.

Methods of preparation and administration: Soak both red and white fleeceflower roots in the water in which rice has been washed for 3-4 days, and remove the skin with a bamboo knife. Put them together with black beans layer by layer, one layer for fleeceflower roots and another layer for black beans, and steam them. When the black beans are done, replace them with new black beans and steam them in the same way. After the fleeceflower roots are steamed nine times this way, dry them and pestle them into powder. Skin both the red and white Indian breads, wash them clean and pound them into pieces. Soak and mix them with human milk, dry them and pestle them into powder. Remove the seedlings from the two-toothed achyranthes, soak it in wine for one day and steam it together with the fleeceflower roots from the seventh time steaming. Dry it and pestle it into powder. Soak the dodder seeds until they sprout, soak them in wine for one night, dry them and pestle them into powder. Stir-bake the scurfpea fruit with black sesame seeds until they smell fragrant, and pestle them into powder. Mix all the powders together and make pellets with honey the size of a Chinese parasol seed.

Take 20 pellets at a time, three times a day, with warm rice wine in the morning, ginger soup at noon, and lightly salted water in the evening. It nourishes the kidneys, strengthens the bones, invigorates the function of the brain and marrow, and improves sexual performance. It helps cure early whitening of hair and beard, dizziness, sore muscles and bones, sore waist and knees, neurasthenia, male sterility, and failure of sexual function. This recipe provides a good combination of medicines. It is nutritious and is good for use by middle-aged and old people over a long period of time. Emperor Shizong of the Ming Dynasty gave birth to several princes by taking these pellets.

Qinggong Shoutao Balls (*Remarks by Qing Dynasty Court Physicians*)

Ingredients: Ginseng, Danggui (Chinese angelica root), Yizhiren (sharpleaf galangal seed), Dashengdi (large rehmannia root), Gouqi (wolfberry fruit), Tianmendong (asparagus root), and walnut kernels.

Methods of preparation and administration: Pestle all the ingredients together into powder and make them into balls with honey, each ball weighing 6 g. Take one ball at a time with warm water, every morning and evening. It improves feminine energy, strengthens masculine energy, and prolongs life. It also helps cure deficiency of both Yin and Yang *qi*, insufficiency of *qi* and blood, dizziness, tinnitus, dacryorrhea, fatigue, sore waist, and increased excretion of urine at night.

Points for attention when using any of these tonics:

First of all, know your own physical condition and the nature of your illness. For example, whether you are deficient in vital energy or blood, whether it is a deficiency of Yin *qi* or Yang *qi*, vital essence of the heart or of the lungs, or of the liver or spleen. Only when you have a clear understanding of these conditions can you take the right medicine to cure your illness. It is better to go to a traditional Chinese doctor for medical advice before making a decision.

8. Medicated diet

Medicated diet means blending traditional Chinese medicine with food to make medicated food for the prevention and treatment of illness, the improvement of health and the prolonging of life. It is believed that in primitive society, medicine and food were the same thing. In the long process of searching for food, man found many drugs accidentally. At that time, man gathered the roots, stems, leaves and fruits of plants, and insects, animals and fish for food, not like the food people have today. There was originally no knowledge to distinguish between edibles and non-edibles. Experience was gradually gained, and with it came knowledge of what could and could not be eaten. This was the origin of the drugs. There is a story about "Shen Nong tasting a hundred herbs and meeting with 70 poisonous substances in a day" in ancient times. This symbolizes the historical process of how our forefathers discovered the medicinal uses of plants, and gradually accumulated traditional Chinese medicines.

In traditional Chinese medicine, some drugs can be used as food, and some food can be used as drugs to cure illnesses, such as Chinese yam, lotus seeds, dried longan pulp, almonds, jingjie (schizonepeta), coriander, ginger, Chinese dates, bee honey, haws, pear and water chestnuts. They are both foods and drugs, and can both nourish the body and cure illnesses. Medicated diets are designed on the basis of the characteristics of Chinese medicines. Following are recipes for some traditional, common and effective Chinese medicated diets:

(1) Medicated porridges: Add a suitable amount of soup or water

to the medicated foodstuffs. First boil them over a high fire and then cook them over a low flame until the food melts and the soup or water thickens. Medicated porridges are easily absorbed and digested and are particularly good for middle-aged and old people.

Lotus leaf porridge (*Guide to Dietetic Treatment*): Take one fresh lotus leaf, add water 750 ml, boil it for 10 minutes, remove the lotus leaf, add 60 g round-grained non-glutinous rice and appropriate amount of white granulated sugar or crystal sugar, cook slowly over a low flame until the rice grains melt and the liquid becomes thick and sticky. This can be used for breakfast and supper, and it helps cure headache, dizziness, hypertension, obesity, high blood lipids, and arteriosclerosis.

Ginseng porridge (*Dietetic Mirror Materia Medica*): Ginseng (powdered) 3 g, round-grained non-glutinous rice 60 g, crystal sugar. Put them together in an earthenware pot and add 750 ml water to make porridge. Eat for breakfast and supper in autumn and winter to help improve vital energy, nourish the five internal organs, and resist senile decline. It is a good food for the middle-aged and elderly who are physically weak, suffer from a deficiency of energy in the five internal organs, bad appetite, insomnia, poor memory, and failing sexual function. It is not suitable for middle-aged and old people who are strong-bodied or who suffer from the flaming-up of fire due to a deficiency of Yin energy or in the hot summer weather. Avoid eating turnips and drinking tea while taking this porridge.

Chinese yam porridge (*Saqian's Experience Prescriptions*): Powdered yam 50 g (fresh yam 100 g) and round-grained non-glutinous rice 50 g. Cook them together with water to make porridge, and eat for breakfast and supper. It reinforces the spleen and stomach and nourishes the lungs and kidneys. It also helps cure deficiency in the spleen, diarrhea, consumption, cough, poor appetite, and fatigue.

Lilyturf root porridge: Lilyturf root 30 g, round-grained non-glutinous rice 50 g, and crystal sugar 20 g. Cook them together with water to make porridge, and eat for breakfast. This moistens the lungs and clears the heart of internal heat. It also helps cure deficiency and dryness in the lungs, cough, haemoptysis, consumption, fever with dysphoria, insufficiency of Yin energy in the stomach, febrile disease, deficiency of fluid, and dry throat and thirst.

Eight-treasure porridge (traditional Chinese food): According to Chinese custom, families eat porridge for breakfast on the eighth day of the twelfth lunar month. Since this porridge is made of eight nutritious ingredients, it is called "eight-treasure porridge." However, the porridge is not eaten only on the eighth day of the twelfth month, but also on other days. It is especially good for the middle-aged and elderly all year round. The eight treasures are Qianshi (euryale seed), Yiyiren (job's-tears seed), Baibiandou (white hyacinth bean), lotus seed, Chinese yam, red dates, longan pulp and lily. Use 6 g each, water and boil them for 40 minutes. Add round-grained non-glutinous rice 150 g, and continue to cook until they melt in the mouth. Add both white sugar and brown sugar, 20 g each, and mix them well. Divide the porridge equally for three breakfasts. This helps cure weakness, fatigue, edema caused by deficiency, diarrhea, insomnia, diabetes, and cough.

Tremella porridge (*Liu Juanzi's Devil Left Recipes*): Yin'er (tremella, also called white fungus) 10 g. Soak in water for four hours, then wash clean. First cook five Chinese dates and 60 g round-grained non-glutinous rice with water for 30 minutes, then add tremella and crystal sugar, and continue cooking for another 10 minutes until it becomes porridge. Eat for breakfast and supper. This replenishes Yin energy to relieve the lungs from dryness, making up for deficiency and strengthening the spleen. It also helps middle-aged and elderly people overcome physical weakness, anaemia, pulmonary tuberculosis, coronary heart disease, chronic heptitis, allergic purpura, habitual constipation, bleeding piles, and arteriosclerosis.

Milkvetch root porridge (*Medical Talks from the Deserted House*):

Huangqi (milkvetch root) 20 g. Boil in water for 40 minutes and remove the dregs. Add 60 g round-grained non-glutinous rice to make porridge. Eat on an empty stomach for breakfast. This replenishes the vital energy, relieves swelling, strengthens body resistance, and stops sweating. It also helps prevent cold, and improves immunity and the functioning of the cardiovascular system, lungs, and kidneys.

Wolfberry fruit porridge (*The Peaceful Holy Benevolent Prescriptions*): Gouqi (wolfberry fruit) 15 g, and rice 50 g. Cook them to make porridge, and eat on an empty stomach in the morning. This nourishes the liver and kidneys, replenishes the semen, and improves eyesight. It also helps cure deficiency of Yin energy in the liver and kidneys, dizziness, poor eye sight, hypertension, and diabetes.

Indian bread porridge (*Compendium of Materia Medica*): Baifuling (powdered white Indian bread) 30 g, and round-grained non-glutinous rice 100 g. Cook them together to make porridge and eat on an empty stomach for breakfast. This strengthens the spleen and maintains tranquility, promotes the excretion of urine and relieves swelling. It also helps cure deficiency in the spleen, diarrhea, neurasthenia, and obesity.

Milk porridge (*Compendium of Materia Medica*): Use rice 100 g and cook it with water into porridge, then add cow milk, or sheep milk, or horse milk 500 g, and white sugar 30 g. Boil it again. Eat for breakfast and supper. This will make up for deficiency, nourish the heart and lungs, remove the poison caused by heat, relieve diabetes, and promote smooth the large intestines. It also helps cure consumption, deficiency of the lungs, and cough in the middle-aged and old people.

Cistanche porridge (*Treatise on the Nature of Drugs*): Roucongrong (cistanche) 12 g. Put it into an earthenware pot, add water and cook it for about 40 minutes until it becomes soft. Remove the dregs and keep the liquid, add rice 60 g to make porridge. Eat once a day, for breakfast or supper. It will moisten dryness to facilitate the smooth passage of food through the intestines, and nourish the kidneys to invigorate masculine energy. It also helps cure deficiency of Yang energy, constipation, impotence, and early emission.

Rehmannia root porridge (*The Heart Mirror for Food and Clothing*): Use rice 60 g to make porridge, add bee honey and Shengdi (rehmannia juice use 60 g fresh rehmannia root and pound it to extract the juice), mix them well and eat on an empty stomach. This will invigorate the heart, facilitate the excretion of urine, and stop bleeding. It also helps in treating diabetes, rheumatism, rheumatoid arthritis, hematemesis, hematochezia, nose bleeding, and swollen and sore throat.

Walnut porridge (*Sea Collection of Proven Recipes*): Six large walnuts. Shell the walnuts, remove the nuts and put them in 60 g rice, and add water to make porridge. Eat on an empty stomach in the morning or evening, once a day. It will moisten the lungs to resolve phlegm, nourish the kidneys, and relieve asthma. It also helps cure deficiency of the kidneys, lumbago, deficiency of the lungs cough, early whitening of hair, neurasthenia, and renal obstruction.

Lotus root porridge (*Old Folk's Common Talk*): Fresh lotus root 100 g (remove the knots and skin, wash it clean and cut it into slices), round-grained non-glutinous rice 60 g and white granulated sugar 10 g. Cook them together in an earthenware pot and eat for breakfast or supper, once a day. This will strengthen the spleen and regulate the stomach, nourish the blood and stop diarrhea. It also helps cure the senile weakness, poor appetite, sticky and loose stools, dry mouth, and excessive thirst.

(2) Medicated cakes: Medicated cakes are soft and spongy cakes made of rice flour, powdered drugs, and white sugar and cut into large pieces. As they are easily digested and have the effect of nourishing body parts and curing illnesses, they are good for the middle-aged and older people. In the *Compendium of Materia Medica* medicated cakes are described as "having the effect of nourishing the spleen, stomach, and intestines, reinforcing the vital energy, and regulating the stomach."

Spring Snow Cake (*Protection of Vital Energy for Long Life*): Fuling (Indian bread), Chinese yam, Qianshi (euryale seeds) and lotus seeds, 120 g each. Pestle them together into powder, add millet flour and glutinous rice flour, 250 g each, white granulated sugar 750 g. and put in water. Mix them into loose granules, then stamp them into the molds. After they are steamed, they are ready to eat. Take around 100 g each time according to your appetite, twice a day. This will strengthen the spleen, regulate the stomach, and relieve diarrhea. It also helps cure deficiency of the spleen, insomnia, poor memory, and increased leukorrhea in women.

Haw jelly (a common traditional food): Fresh, large haws 1,000 g. Wash them clean and steam until they are done. Crush them and remove the skins and stones. Mix the pulp together with round-grained non-glutinous rice flour 500 g and white sugar 500 g to make jelly in the same way as the Spring Snow Cake. Take 30 g each time, once or twice a day. This stimulates digestion and reduces blood lipids. It also helps cure indigestion (especially after eating too much meat) and high blood lipids.

(3) Medicated soup: This is a mixture of chicken, fish, meats,

eggs, and drugs. It is a semi-liquid food cooked with water over slow fire (until the meat melts in the mouth). The solid ingredients in the soup are edible, and the soup is for drinking. The medicated soup not only has nourishing and curing properties, but is also easily absorbed and digested.

Asiabell and milkvetch root chicken soup: Chicken meat 100 g, Dangshen (Asiabell root) 20 g, Huangqi (milkvetch root) 30 g. Put them together with water in an earthenware pot and stew until they are done. Eat the chicken and drink the soup once every five days. This will nourish the spleen and replenish vital energy. It also helps cure ptosis of the internal organs, fatigue, shortness of breath, prolapse of the anus, and chronic sores.

Solomonseal root and pork soup: Huangjing (solomonseal roots) 30 g, and lean pork 100 g. Put them in an earthenware pot, add water and stew over a low flame until the pork is done. Eat the meat and drink the soup to reduce blood lipids and blood sugar, and treat physical weakness, hypertension, and diabetes.

Chinese angelica root, ginger and mutton soup: Lean mutton 100 g, Danggui (angelica root) 20 g and ginger 6 g. Put them together in an earthenware pot and cook with water until the mutton is done. Eat the meat and drink the soup to replenish *qi* and blood, invigorate the kidneys, and improve the sexual performance. It can also help treat physical weakness, deficiency of *qi* and blood, and impotence and early emission.

Gastrodia tuber and black chicken soup: Black chicken meat 100 g and Tianma (gastrodia tuber) 15 g. Cook them with water in an earthenware pot. Eat the chicken meat and drink the soup to replenish *qi* and cure dizziness and numbness in the limbs.

Ginkgo and longan soup: Five ginkgo kernels and longan pulp 10 g and crystal sugar. Cook together and eat it to invigorate the heart and lungs, and cure neurasthenia, cough with phlegm, and increase leukorrhea in women.

(4) Medicated dishes: Medicated dishes are prepared by cooking vegetables, meats, eggs and fish with drugs. They have properties capable of curing illnesses and have therefore become favorite foods among middle-aged and elderly people.

Steamed celery: Fresh celery, 500 g. Wash clean and cut it into pieces. Mix with wheat flour 150 g and steam it until done. Flavor with mashed garlic, table salt and sesame oil to treat hypertension.

Steamed fish: Fresh carp and wax gourd, 100 g each. Put them together in a porcelain bowl with a cover and steam until done. Eat the fish to nourish the kidneys, induce diuresis, and help cure nephritis and edema.

Steamed shepherd's purse: Fresh Qicai (shepherd's purse) 500 g. Prepare it in the same way as steamed celery to reduce blood pressure and stop bleeding. It also helps cure hypertension, nose bleeding, hemoptysis, and womb bleeding during the period of menopause.

(5) Medicinal wine: Please refer to the "Winter" in Chapter One.

(6) Tonic tea: Please refer to the section "Alcoholic beverages, tea and health preservation" in this chapter.

9. Diet for patients in the late stages of febrile diseases

In traditional Chinese medicine, all diseases with or characterized by fever are called "febrile diseases," such as flu, acute tonsillitis, acute bronchitis, acute pneumonia, epidemic meningitis, encephalitis B, and all other fever-producing diseases. As fever causes the loss of saliva, even if the patient recovers from his illness and the fever goes down, he may still suffer from saliva deficiency, resulting in dry throat, irritability, feverishness in the palms and soles, and deficiency of saliva on the tongue. In this case, the patient should take light food to replenish Yin *qi*, food such as thin rice porridge, Chinese yam porridge, rehmannia porridge, lilyturf root porridge, lotus root porridge, or milk porridge. He can also eat fresh fruit and vegetables such as water chestnuts, pears, sugar cane, carrots, tomatoes, and watermelon to help replenish Yin *qi* and produce saliva.

10. Diet for the elderly

Diseases particular to old people include atherosclerosis, hypertension, coronary heart disease, chronic senile bronchitis, diabetes, hypertrophy of the prostate gland, rheumatoid arthritis, and tumors. The following are suggested diets for those suffering from diseases common to the elderly.

(1) High blood lipids, coronary heart disease, and hypertension: The best staple foods for sufferers of these diseases are a mixed diet of rice, millet, corn flour, wheat flour, and bean flour. The non-staple foods should include celery, onion, wild rice stem, bitter gourd, shepherd's purse, cucumber, kelp, laver, turnip, bean sprouts, and garlic. The best oils include soybean oil, sunflower seed oil, rape oil, sesame seed oil, and peanut oil. Avoid eating foods with a high cholesterol content such as animal fat, internal organs, brains, and egg yolks. Eat less salt and sugar. It is advisable to eat a proper amount of lean meat, fish and egg whites. You can also choose, from among the medicated diets, lotus leaf porridge, tremella porridge, wolfberry fruit porridge, haw cake, steamed celery, and steamed shepherd's purse as described in the preceding sections.

(2) Diabetes: In the literature of traditional Chinese medicine, diabetes is known as the "disease of consumption and thirst." It is characterized by eating more, drinking more, and urinating more.

Moderation in eating and drinking is basic for treating diabetes.

A common diabetic can improve his condition by using the diet therapy, but a serious diabetic should use diet therapy to supplement medical treatment with drugs to achieve satisfactory results. Diabetics should strictly control the amount of staple foods, fruits, and sugar they eat. They should eat more vegetables that are abundant in vitamins and cellulose and are low in carbohydrates such as celery, shepherd's purse, bitter gourd, cucumber, pumpkin, bean sprouts, and onion and garlic. Among fruits, they should eat pomegranate, haws, and Chinese yam. They should also eat foods containing more protein such as soybeans and products made of soybeans, lean meat, and eggs. Many Chinese herbal drugs that help reduce blood sugar are recommended for frequent use as medicated foods, such as Chinese yam, haws, ginseng, milkvetch root, solomonseal rhizome, wolfberry, Indian bread, lilyturf root, rehmannia rhizome, kudzuvine root and fleeceflower root. The "Qian Jin Bu Lao Pellet" described above and patent Chinese drugs such as Yu Quan Wan, Xiao Ke Wan and Maiwei Dihuang Wan all have good curative effects for diabetes.

(3) Obesity: Obesity is overweight caused by the over-accumulation of fats in the human body. The normal weight for adults can be calculated in the following simple way: The standard weight for a man: (kilograms) = height (centimeters)-100, and that for a woman, (kilograms) = height (centimeters)-102.

Obese people are in danger of coronary heart disease, hypertension, diabetes, fatty liver, gallbladder stones, and gout. So old people especially should pay attention to preventing obesity.

Prevention of obesity is usually called "weight reduction" today and was known as "making the body lighter" in ancient times. Temperance in eating and drinking is paramount. It is essential to eat low-calorie foods, eat less sugar, fatty meat and fried foods, and eat more vegetables, fruits and lean meat. The ancients advocated the theory of "eating less to prolong life," and especially stressed that "the stomach should never be full after supper." If you do not overeat, keep your weight constant, and have a normal heart, you may then enjoy a longer life. The lotus leaf porridge and Fuling (Indian bread) porridge already described have certain properties for weight control. One prescription of controlling weight is the following: Haws, Fuling (Indian bread), Zexie (water-plantain tuber), Maiya (germinated barley), Caojueming (cassia seeds) and tea leaves, 100 g each. Pestle them into powder. Use 6-10 g each time and pour boiled water on it for oral administration, 15 days for a course of treatment. Persist in drinking this tea and your weight will be reduced.

(4) Chronic bronchitis: Chronic bronchitis sufferers often have deficiency of *qi* in the lungs, spleen, and kidneys. As for diet therapy these patients should choose foods that help strengthen the spleen, regulate the flow of *qi* and nourish the lungs and kidneys. Such foods are turnips, tangerines, loquats, pears, lily, lotus seeds, Chinese dates, almonds, Chinese yam, walnuts, bee honey, water chestnuts and sugar cane. Changchun Yishou Pellets, Qianjin Bulao Pellets, yam porridge, lilyturf root porridge, eight-treasure porridge, walnut porridge and ginkgo and longan pulp porridge are all good for you, depending on your condition.

(5) Chronic gastritis: gastric and duodenal ulcers: These are all called "stomachache" in traditional Chinese medicine, and are a common complaint among old people. If you have one of these conditions, you must first of all give up smoking and eat food rich in protein, vitamins and minerals. It is advisable to take soft rice, porridge, and wheaten foods, and eat less, but more often. Fish, lean meat, eggs and soybean products also should be taken more often. Avoid eating fried, cold, pungent, raw and hard foods. Ginseng porridge, milkvetch root porridge, eight- treasure porridge, and Yannian Yishou Pellets are suggested. The following recipe is

also suggested for stomach ailments: Fish bladder 500 g, cuttlefish bone and the bulb of fritillary, 300 g each, Baiji (bletilla tuber), and Sanqishen (notoginseng), 30 g each, Danggui (Chinese angelica root), white peony root, Chaihu (thorowax root), Fuling (Indian bread), Baizhu (bighead atractylodes), bitter orange, sandalwood, Gaoliangjiang (galangal rhizome), Xiangfu (flatsedge tuber), Guangmuxiang (costus root), green tangerine peel, tangerine peel and Suye (perilla seed leaf), 20 g each. Pestle them together into fine powder. Take 4 g each time after pouring liquid on it, three times a day, and even better with thin millet porridge or warm boiled water.

Constipation: Constipation is another problem commonly found among the aging. Because these folks gradually become deficient in vital energy and blood, they have greater difficulty moistening the stools, causing dry stools and making it difficult to eliminate the feces from the bowels. In this case, they should eat foods with more cellulose to stimulate the peristalsis of the intestinal passages. Such foods are fresh vegetables, fruits, coarse grains and beans. Spinach, carrots, onions, and bananas also may have an effect. Also, bee honey helps to moisten feces. Use 30-50 ml honey and pour boiled water on it to make honey tea. Caojueming (cassia seed) is good for reducing blood lipids and blood pressure, and relieving constipation. Pestle 15 g cassia seeds into powder to make tea. It both moisten the stools and treats hypertension and high blood lipids. Tremella porridge, milk porridge and cistanche porridge all have good effect in curing constipation, and can be taken daily.

Constipation sufferers should not drink alcoholic beverages or eat pungent foods.

Chapter Four
Regular Life

The physicians of ancient China regarded a "regular life" as an important condition for a long life. People who take care of their health arrange their daily work and rest schedule on a scientific basis of seasonal changes in climate and observe them consciously. A regular life can ensure the vigorous growth of vital energy in the kidneys, keep you in good health, improve immunity and increase resistance to disease. If your life is irregular, it may harm your health, shorten your life and you may face an early decline.

1. Cultivate good living habits

Good living habits include, conforming to seasonal changes and making a reasonable arrangements of your life. Details have been described for the first aspect in the "Seasonal Methods" in this book, and no more words will be given in this chapter. Here we will deal with the regular life.

Modern medical research demonstrates that a regular life is needed for a long life. A regular life enables the tissues and organs of the human body to acquire the proper stimulation and work rhythmically in the central nervous system. Of the body's rhythms, the heartbeat and breathing are most evident and easily felt. A regular life maintains these rhythms and are good for the rhythmical activities of the other organs. If life is irregular, this rhythmical movement will be disturbed, harming the health and even life.

A regular life is good for the formation of conditional reflexs, and this is likewise beneficial to good health and long life. Take the cerebral cortex as an example. If one goes to bed and gets up on a fixed schedule every day, and if things go on like this for a long time, a conditional reflex will be formed. When it is time to sleep, the cerebral cortex will become inhibited, and one becomes sleepy and falls to sleep right after going to bed. When it is time to get up, the cerebral cortex becomes excited, waking one up from sleep. Then one is vigorous and energetic and able to work efficiently. If life is irregular, the rhythms of the cerebral cortex are disrupted. The intestines and stomach are another example. If you eat regularly every day, a conditional reflex is formed. However, if the meals are taken irregularly the gastric and intestinal functions are confused, and gastric and intestine diseases like indigestion, stomachache, abdominal pains and diarrhea may occur.

The "theory of directing *qi* (vital energy)" in traditional Chinese medicine includes "time biology" and the "theory of the biological clock." The "theory of directing *qi*" holds that there is regular movement of *qi* and blood in the human body, just like the movement of celestial bodies. The movement of *qi* and blood in the body and the movement of the celestial bodies are closely related. *Qi*, the vital energy, and blood just like a clock, moves nonstop day and night and is influenced by the movement of celestial bodies. This theory has become the cornerstone for "time biology," "time therapeutics" and "the theory of the biological clock." In other words, the modern "theory of the biological clock" has emerged from the womb of the "theory of directing *qi*" in traditional Chinese medicine. If the "biological clock" of the body is to work rhythmically and regularly, life must be regular and rhythmical. Only when the "biological clock" works regularly and rhythmically is it possible to achieve the goal of eliminating diseases, keeping in good health and prolonging life.

2. Sleeping hygiene

Sleep is vital to the existence of mankind, the protective agent of the nervous system. A man may be on a hunger strike for weeks, but will have great difficulty if he goes a week without any sleep.

Specialists in ancient China attached great importance to the influence of sleep on long life, and used sleep as an important method to keep themselves in good health. The medical book *Ten Questions,* unearthed from a Han Dynasty tomb at Mawangdui in Changsha, holds that sleep can promote digestion and the distribution of the medicinal power. Li Yu, in the Qing Dynasty, wrote in his *Collected Works of an Old Man with a Bamboo Hat*: "The secret of health preservation is, first of all, sleep. It can regenerate the semen, improve health, invigorate the spleen and stomach, and strengthen bones and muscles." *The Yellow Emperor's Canon of Medicine* and other ancient classics also hold that one should go to bed late and get up early in spring and summer, and go to bed early and get up late in autumn and winter. The time to get up should not be earlier than when the cock crows, nor later than sunrise.

It is a good habit to take a nap at noon. It is even more important for the middle-aged and old people because afternoon naps help improve immunity, prevent coronary heart disease, hypertension, gastritis and dementia, and prolong life. Investigation shows that those with the habit of taking naps after lunch have better immunity than those who do not nap. They should take naps for about 30 minutes after lunch, and rise slowly.

During sleep, all activities of the tissue slow down to reaccumulate energy.

As to posture, it is the best to lie on your side. People in ancient times held that one should not lie with the head toward the north, because the north is Yin in Yin. The head should not face north so that the cold Yin *qi* does not hurt the body's vital *qi*.

Physicians in ancient China also summed up their experience as the ten avoidances for sleep: One, avoid lying on the back while sleeping, because in this posture the body is straight and not relaxed, the muscles are tense, and the hands are easily placed on the chest, giving rise to nightmares and affecting breathing and the heartbeat. One should lie on the side with knees bent, in this way the vital essence and energy will not be hindered. When waking up, one should stretch in order to promote the circulation of *qi* and blood. Two, avoid anxiety. When going to sleep, do not worry or think too much, but keep calm. Cai Jitong of the Song Dynasty meant exactly the same thing when he wrote in his *Secret of Sleep*: "When going to sleep, relax your mind before falling asleep." Three, avoid anger. Anger causes disorder in the circulation of *qi* and blood, leading to insomnia or illness. Four, avoid overeating before going to bed. If one overeats, the burden on the intestines and stomach is increased, affecting sleep. The instruction in *Questions and Answers* that "indigestion disturbs sleep" is truly the wise remark of an experienced person. Five, avoid talking too much before going to bed, because too much talk keeps one excited, thus affecting sleep and causing insomnia. Six, avoid sleeping while facing the light. Facing the light while sleeping distracts one's mind, making it difficult to fall asleep. Seven, avoid sleeping with the mouth open. Sleeping at night with the mouth closed is a good way to preserve the primordial *qi*. Breathing with the mouth open is bad for health. It also subjects the lungs to stimulation by cold air and dust, thus causing illness. Eight, avoid sleeping with the head covered. Sleeping with the head covered under the quilt makes it difficult for one to breathe as the air under the quilt is foul, and therefore unhealthy. Nine, avoid sleeping in the wind. Wind is the first and foremost factor causing many diseases. It is always changing direction capriciously and is always likely to attack the human body and cause illness. When one sleeps, "the Yang *qi* (masculine energy) stays inside." The Yang *qi* resists attack from outside evils, but if it returns to inside the body, the resistance of the body is weakened, thus subjecting it to attack by the wind and evils. Therefore, be sure not to sleep in the wind. Ten, avoid sleeping with the head against the stove. Sleeping with the head against the stove, one is likely to be attacked by the heat, making the head heavy and the eyes red, or causing boils, carbuncles, or cold.

Along with these ten avoidances, one should not drink strong tea, coffee or cocoa before going to bed, because these beverages have stimulants that disturb sleep and may cause insomnia. Middle-aged and older people should sleep on soft and comfortable beds, and their bedrooms should be free of wind and strong light. The quilts should be soft and warm and the pillows neither too high nor too low. Patients may use pillows stuffed with medicinal herbs. Those with hypertension or those suffering from headache or dizziness can use pillows with chrysanthemum, cassia, mung beans, and other medicinal herbs. Insomnia sufferers can use pillows filled with rush or magnet powder. Sufferers of nasosinusitis with pus can use pillows filled with the powder of Baizhi (dahurian angelica root) or Xinxi (magnolia flower). Sufferers of glaucoma can put the coarse powder of Xiakucao (selfheal spike), lotus leaf, Baizhi (dahurian angelica root) or Caojueming (herbal cassia) in their pillows. Patients with headache induced by cold can put steamed Wuzhuyu (evodia fruit) in their pillows and those with internal heat and pain in the ears can put heated salt in the pillows.

In order to have a good sleep, it is advisable to wash the feet in warm water before going to bed so to promote the circulation of vital energy and blood.

Too much sleep can also be bad for your health. *Questions and Answers* says that "long sleep harms the vital energy." Sleep must be proper, it should not be too little, nor too much. Investigations have shown that the mortality rate for people with ten or more hours of sleep a night is 80 percent higher than that for those with eight hours of sleep a night. Eight hours a night is enough sleep for people under 70. Those between 70 and 90 should sleep nine hours, and those over 90 should sleep 10-12 hours a night.

3. Housing hygiene

In ancient China, great importance was attached to the selection of the location of a house. It was believed that location had a close bearing on the health and long life of the occupants, the prosperity of the family, and on whether or not a family member would obtain an official position or make a fortune. Before a new house was built, a geomancer was often invited to select the location. A good location was called "a treasured location of good *feng shui* (wind and water)." The nucleus of *feng shui* is a branch of knowledge indicating how to select and arrange the living enviornment. It includes the selection of the geographical location for a house, whether the topographical conditions can satisfy the occupants of the new house psychologically and physiologically, and general features such as the use and transformation of the natural surroundings, the direction the house faces, and its height, size, entrance, road, water supply and drainage. *Feng shui*, in essence, involves geology, meteorology, hydrology, architecture, psychology and environmental protection. *Feng shui* is believed to influence human health. For example, the direction of the magnetic force line of the earth, the direction of the flow of the underground water, and the direction of the flow of the rivers, the direction of the wind all have an influence. If the surroundings are not good and the direction of the house is not desirable, dire consequences may, in time, ensue. This coincides with the traditional Chinese medical theory of human adaptation to the natural environment. This theory holds that man and nature are closely linked together, that man is inseparable from nature, and that the natural environment and the movement of the celestial bodies have a bearing on human health. *Feng shui* has at times been misused by the witches and sorcerers and coated with mystical and superstitious colors. And we are not going to say any more on this point.

Ancient Chinese physicians developed the scientific part of the theory, and advanced the theory of "environmental medical science." They noted: "Food, drink and living places are the sources of illnesses." They clearly pointed out that ill-conceived housing was one of the important factors generating disease, and that housing should be arranged reasonably and with appropriate living conditions. What are appropriate living conditions? It can be summed up in the following points:

(1) Quiet and beautiful living environment: Houses should be built on high, dry, clean and hygienic places to keep the dwellers in good health and prolong their life. If the houses are located in damp, dirty and filthy low-lying places, the dwellers will fall sick all the year round and perhaps even die early. Therefore, the ancient people attached great importance to the selection of housing locations and living environment. The living environment selected by ancient physicians were all very quiet and beautiful. For example, Sun Simiao, the famous Tang Dynasty physician, had his house built by a beautiful hill and water, and planted trees and flowers to spend his late years, and lived 101 years.

(2) Good housing structure: Houses should be properly built with a good structure to benefit health and prolong life. Sun Simiao

said: "All rooms must be well built with no cracks to allow the wind to come in." Chen Zhi said: "The bedroom must be always clean and elegant. It should be open in summer and closed tightly in winter. The sleeping bed should not be high or broad, it should be one-third smaller than the regular bed. The mattress must be soft and flat. Screens should be placed on three sides to prevent cold wind." This means that the bedrooms should be warm in winter and cool in summer, and windproof and dampproof.

People in ancient China were very particular about the direction of the house, the position of the bed, the light in the bedroom, the height of the house, and the opening and closing of the windows. For example, the book *Tian Yin Zi on Health Building* says: "What is a good living place? It is not a magnificent and large house with well-furnished beds. It should face the south with the head toward the east when sleeping. There should be harmony between Yin and Yang, half dark and half bright. The house should not be too high, or it will have too much light and Yang. Neither should it be too low, or it will have too much dankness and Yin. When there is too much light, it does damage to the *hun* (the Yang spirit). When there is too much darkness, it does damage to the *po* (the Yin spirit). The *hun* of the human being is Yang while the *po* is Yin. If both the *hun* and *po* are hurt, there is illness. In the house where I live, I have a curtain in front and a screen in the rear. When it is too bright, I put down the curtain to reduce the light inside. If it is too dark, I raise the curtain to let in more light. Refresh the mind internally and please the eyes externally. When both the mind and eyes are sound, nothing happens to the human body."

Moreover, people in ancient China also attached great importance to the layout of the house. They often built houses into courtyards of a certain shape so that people could enjoy the outdoor sunshine, air, flowers, trees, and other natural elements.

(3) Clean and hygienic living places: Clean houses help reduce the occurrence of disease and improve the health of the dwellers. The hygiene standards for living places are:

Temperature: The most appropriate room temperature is 16 = 24 degrees Centigrade, slightly higher in summer, between 21 = 32 degrees Centigrade.

Humidity: The relative room humidity should be 50-60 percent, but not less than 35 percent in winter and no higher than 70 percent in summer.

Ventilation: The air should be well circulated inside the rooms. Both the front and back windows should be opened to allow the smooth circulation of air, but the velocity of the air flow should not be too high. It is good enough just to keep the room well ventilated. Because traditional Chinese medicine holds that "wind is the root source of all diseases."

Brightness: If the light is poor, it gives the dweller a sense of depression, loneliness and listlessness, and causes fatigue. If the light is too strong, it makes the dweller irritable or even dizzy. Appropriate light keeps people vigorous and broad-minded. The rooms should have transparent glass windows for the natural light to penetrate through. The colors of the walls and ceiling should be soft, light yellow, light blue, light orange, light apple green or other light but elegant colors, depending on your own liking.

Quiet: Quiet in the house is beneficial to health. Noise not only hurts the ears and affects sleep, but also may creat functional disorders of the internal organs. Therefore, it is important to keep the room noiseless, quiet and comfortable. If the house fronts the street or a factory, the doors and windows must be closed tight against the noisy disturbance or equipped with thick window curtains with a good soundproof effect or other soundproof devices.

Tidiness: The furniture in the bedroom should be as simple and practical as possible. It should be kept clean, neat and tidy. There should be space for indoor activity. It is advisable to hang some paintings, calligraphies or landscape pictures. Handicraft articles or potted landscapes may be put on the bookshelf or desk for show. All this is intended to create a pleasant atmosphere.

4. Cleansing hygiene

Good personal hygiene is essential for maintaining health, dignity and department.

(1) Wash face, hair and hands: In addition to washing their faces every day middle-aged and older people should rub their faces to stimulate the circulation of blood and to keep the skin tender and crease free. It is also essential to wash the hair every five to seven days. This helps protect the hair and keep it black and shining. It also helps stimulate the nerves to improve the physique and the brain. Attention should be paid to the following points in washing the hair and face:

The temperature and cleanliness of the water: The water should be clean, hygienic and pollution-free, and the temperature should be neither too high nor too low. It is good enough if you fell warm and comfortable. It is best to use warm tap water to wash the face and hair to ensure cleanliness, freshness and comfort.

Towel and toilet soap: Make sure that only one person uses one basin and one towel. In other words, both the basin and towel should be used exclusively. Toilet soap should be used, not laundry soap, because laundry soap contains more sodium and is irritating and harmful to the skin. Toilet soap contains less sodium, and is neutral and suitable for use.

To ensure that the hair remains soft, black, and shiny, it is advisable to use 60 g of Heshouwu (fleeceflower root) boiled in water for 60 minutes, remove the residue and use the liquid or tea liquid to wash the hair after shampoo.

After hair washing, be sure not to catch cold to avoid facial paralysis and cerebral blood vessel diseases.

The hands are easily subjected to pollution and are therefore a major channel for spreading germs and causing disease. It is a good habit to wash hands before meal and after shit.

The skin of middle-aged and elderly people is often dry and easily chaped, especially in winter, because secretion from their sebaceous glands and sweat glands has decreased. Therefore, after washing, they should apply some moisturizer, such as face cream, cream with pearl powder or 30 percent glycerine.

(2) Rinsing the mouth and brushing the teeth: Gargling helps remove food particles and reduce germs in the mouth. It is also essential to brush the teeth well. Gargling with warm water and a little salt after meals helps to clean the mouth and kill germs.

Brushing is an effective way to clean the teeth, massage the gums, and protect the surrounding tissue. This requires a good toothbrush and correct brushing technique. When brushing the upper teeth, pull the brush downward and brush the teeth from the top downward, and when brushing the lower teeth, pull the brush upward and brush from the bottom upward. Brush the tongue and the palate surface in the same way, and brush the inner side of the front teeth vertically. Be sure to keep the brush clean after use. A brush should be used exclusively by one person. It is essential to get into the habit of brushing teeth in the morning and evening and gargling after meals. Use regular toothpaste for cleaning the oral cavity and preventing dental diseases, and use medicinal toothpaste for curing periodontisis, gingivitis and tooth allergy.

(3) Bathing: Bathing is a method of washing the body in water or medicinal liquid to prevent and cure diseases.

Baths include cold water baths, hot water baths, warm water baths, mineral water baths, sea water baths, medicinal water baths and steam baths.

Cold water bath: The water temperature is under 20 degrees Centigrade. Bathe in the tub with clean water or take a shower. The length of the bath depends on the physical conditions of the individual. If the water is very cold, bathing time should be no longer than two or three minutes. Use a dry towel to dry the body after the bath, and put on clothes to avoid catching cold. The cold water bath is used to excite the nerves and stimulate the functions of the cardiovascular system, improve the physique, and strengthen adaptability to external surroundings.

Hot water bath: The water temperature is above 39 degrees Centigrade. Usually, it is kept to around 40-45 degrees Centigrade. Bathe 8-10 minutes, two or three times. Dry the body in a warm and fresh room after the bath. Put on clothes when perspiration stops. Hot water baths help dilate the blood vessels, promote blood circulation and improve metabolism, and can also diminish inflammation, ease pain and stop itching. It is also good for rheumatic arthritis, neuralgia, neuritis, chronic poisoning, gout, nephritis, obesity, and skin itch.

Warm water bath: The water temperature is kept to 34-36 degrees Centigrade. This helps keep the nerves calm, relieve the burden on the cardiovascular system, and stop pain. It is also good for hypertension, neurasthenia, and skin itch.

Mineral water bath: Bathe in mineral water in the same way. The temperature of the mineral water is usually high. As the mineral water contains a high concentration of chemicals such as carbonate, sulfate, sulfur, iodine, fluorine, iron, boron, radium, uranium, hydrogen, hydrogen sulfide and sulfur dioxide, it is good for health and medical treatment. It is also good for treating almost all senile diseases, including chronic bronchitis, bronchial asthma, pulmonary emphysema, allergic rhinitis, chronic pharyngitis, gastric spasm, gastric and duodenal ulcers, atrophical gastritis, gastroptosis, hyperacidity, hypoacidity, chronic hepatitis, cholelithiasis, cholecystitis, chronic enteris, phlebitis, hyperthyroidism, gout, diabetes, obesity, chronic prostatitis, and hypertrophy of the prostate.

Sea water bath: Swim or bathe in sea water. Sea water contains various salts of sodium chloride, magnesium chloride, magnesium sulfate, and calcium sulfate, trace elements and gases like oxygen, nitrogen, hydrogen sulfide and carbon dioxide. When these substances stick to the skin, they stimulate the nerve ending so the skin has a slight degree of congestion to improve the circulation of the blood and metabolic function, and improve the function of the reticular endothelial system. The sea water bath helps refresh the body and mind, relax the limbs, and improve metabolism. It is good for curing neurasthenia, obesity, chronic bronchitis, chronic rhinitis, gout, asthma, hypertension, and peripheral vascular diseases.

Sunbath: What are the benefits of sunbathing for the human body?

First of all, the ultraviolet rays of the sun can stimulate the process of excitement, increase the tension of the central nerve and invigorate the internal organs. Moreover, sun rays, the ultraviolet rays in particular, can destroy bacteria. Frequent exposure to sunshine amounts to the sterilization of the entire body and helps strenghten the organisim's immunity. At the same time, ultraviolet rays help to promote the synthesis of Vitamin D inside the body to ensure the normal metabolism of calcium and phosphorus. Sunshine also aids the activities of the heart and lungs, accelerate blood circulation, deepen breathing, and increase vital capacity.

Therefore, those suffering from pulmonary tuberculosis, inhibitive neurosis, cardiovascular disease, arthritis, and chronic enteritis may benefit from sunbathing. People with acute diseases, those with fever, anaemia, skin diseases, excessive fatigue, insomnia, and some pulmonary tuberculosis patients should consult a doctor.

How to sunbathe:

Usually, sunbaths are taken on the beach or at swimming pools. The time can be long or short, first 10 minutes, and then gradually increased to as much as one or two hours. It is best to increase the duration step by step. If you are irradiated for a long time, you should have a break and take a rest in the shade. For medical problems, only the injured or affected parts of the body are exposed to the sun, and the other parts are covered.

What are the points for attention for sunbathing?

Do not take a sunbath after meal or on an empty stomach. It is best to sunbathe some time after you eat and some rest before you eat.

Wear a cap and sunglasses to protect your head and eyes.

Do not fall asleep, smoke or read while sunbathing. You should concentrate on the sunbath.

Rest in the shade after a sunbath and then take a shower.

Generally, 9-11 a.m. and 3-5 p.m. are the best times when the sunlight is not too strong.

If the skin itches, becomes sore, or feels a bit burnt, you should get out of the sun. If you have a headache, feel sick, and suffer from insomnia, arrhythmia or indigestion, you should not take sunbaths.

Medicinal water bath: Prepare the medicinal liquid from traditional Chinese drugs by decoction, and then bathe. This helps treat various diseases. Following are descriptions of the different prescriptions for medicinal baths for some common senile diseases:

Ulcers: Xiakucao (selfheal spike), Jinyinhua (honeysuckle flower), Liujinu (senecio palmatus), and Chishao (red peony root), 30 g each; Pugongying (dandelion) 60 g and Baizhi (dahurian angelia root) 15 g. Decoct them in water and use the liquid for the bath.

Scabies: Use the sulfuric water for the bath.

Skin itching: Fangfeng (saposhnikovia root), Qianghuo (notopterygium root), Jingjie (schizonepeta), Shengdi (rehmannia root), 30 g each; Difuzi (broom cypress fruit), Shechuangzi (cnidium fruit), 50 g each; Chuanwu (Sichuan aconite root), Caowu (wild aconite root), 10 g each, duckweed 100 g. Decoct them in water and use the liquid for the bath in hot water.

Chronic rheumatic and rheumatoid arthritis: Danggui (Chinese angelica root) 15 g, Chuanxiong 30 g, Jixueteng (spatholobus stem) 40 g, Chishao (red peony root) 60 g, Fangfeng (saposhnikovia), Dahuo (pubescent angelica root), Chuanxuduan (Sichuan teasel root), Gouji (cibot rhizome), Bajitian (morinda root), Huluba (fenugreek seed), Chuanniuxi (Sichuan twoteethed achyranthes), and Guizhi (cassia twig), 100 g each. Decoct them in water and take a hot bath with the liquid every day.

Sciatica, pain of the intercostal nerve and neuritis: Danggui (Chinese angelica root), Ruxiang (frankincense), Moyao (myrrh), 20 g each; Honghua (safflower) 30 g, Niuxi (twoteethed achyranthes), black snake, Xuejie (dragon's blood), Ercha (black catechu), 60 g each; Sumu (sappan wood), Chuanxuduan (Sichuan teasel root), Gouji (cibot rhizome), Fangfeng (saposhnikovia), Dahuo (pubescent angelica root), Chuanqianghuo (Sichuan notopterygium), 100 g each; Jixueteng (spatholobus stem) 150 g. Decoct them in water and take a hot bath with the liquid everyday, for 15-30 days.

Gout: Use the same drugs and bathe in the same way as for sciatica.

Injuries from falls, fractures, contusions and strains, sudden sprain of lumbar muscles and pain in the chest when breathing: Danggui

(Chinese angelica root), Tuyuan (ground beetles), Danpi (root bark of tree peony), Fuzi (prepared aconite lateral root), Ruxiang (frankincense), Moyao (myrrh), Ercha (catechu) 20g each; Chuanxiong, Honghua (safflower), peach kernel, Chishao (red peony root), Guizhi (cassia twig), Xuejie (dragon's blood), Zirantong (pyrite), Chuanxuduan (Sichuan teasel root), 30 g each; Zelan (bugleweed), Gusiubu (drynaria rhizome), 60 g each. Decoct them in water and take a warm water bath, once a day.

Chronic nephritis: Huangqi (milkvetch), Fangfeng (saposhnikovia), Chuanxuduan (Sichuan teasel root), Gouji (cibot rhizome), Huluba (fenugreek seed), Guizhi (cassia twig), Cangzhu (atractylodes rhizome), and Baizhu (bighead atractylodes rhizome), 60 g each; Zexie (water plantain tuber) 45 g, Fuping (duckweed), Rendongteng (honeysuckle stem), Dongguapi (wax-gourd peel), 100 g each. Decoct them with water and take a hot bath with the liquid everyday.

Obesity: Wax-gourd peel, Fuling (Indian bread peel), 500 g each; Mugua (flowering-quince fruit) 300 g. Decoct them with water and take a hot bath with the liquid. Be sure to eat and drink moderately.

Cirrhosis with ascites: Mangxiao (sodium sulfate), Dahuang (rhubarb), Gansui (kansui root), Qianxiuzi (pharbitis seed), 50 g each. Decoct them with water. Bathe the entire body when the temperature of the liquid is raised to 40 degrees Centigrade, once a day.

Constipation: Bathe in the same way as for cirrhosis with ascites.

Dropsy: Mahuang (ephedra), Qianghuo (notopterygium), Cangzhu (atractylodes rhizome), Chaihu (thorowax root), Zisu (perilla), Jingjie (schizonepeta), Fangfeng (saposhnikovia), Niubangzi (burdock fruit), Rendongteng (honeysuckle stem), willow twig and scallion stalk, 60 g each. Decoct them with water. When the temperature of the medicinal liquid is raised to 40 degrees Centigrade, bathe the entire body until it sweats, once a day.

When middle-aged and elderly people take baths they should adjust the water temperature and the bathing time according to their own physical condition. The temperature should not be too high and bathing time should not be too long for those who are very weak or who suffer from cardiovascular diseases. They should stop bathing as soon as they feel dizzy, sick, oppressed in the chest, or fidgety, and lie down in a warm, fresh and quiet room.

The interval between baths depends on the seasonal changes and personal needs. Take one bath a day in summer, every two or three days in spring and autumn, and once a week in winter. If using a medicinal bath to treat diseases, take one bath a day.

Middle-aged and elderly people should not take baths when hungry or right after meals. This may easily cause cerebral haemorrhage or myocardial infarction. Be sure to avoid wind and catching cold after baths. Traditional Chinese medicine holds that "wind is the first and foremost factor causeing many diseases." As the pores are open after a bath, the cold air easily enters through the pores, causing diseases.

(4) Wash feet: Washing the feet not only helps remove the dust, sweat and dead skin from the feet and the stinking smell, but also stimulates the circulation of the blood, removes fatigue, promotes sleep and cures insomnia and emission. According to traditional Chinese theory, foot washing "elevates the spleen Yang and prevents collapse in spring, removes pathogenic dampness in summer, moistens the lungs in autumn, and warms the elixir field in winter." In recent years, Chinese medical scientists have also observed the corresponding reflecting areas of the internal organs on the feet on the basis of the traditional Chinese medicinal theory of meridians. If one massages the toes and soles while washing the feet, this can help prevent and cure many diseases. The thumbs are the channels

of the liver and spleen meridians, which help to soothe the liver and invigorate the function of the spleen and increase appetite. The fourth toe is the channel of the gallbladder meridian, which helps to prevent constipation and hypochondriac pain. The little toe is the channel of the urinary bladder meridian, which helps to treat frequent urination, ischuria and continuous dripping of urine. The soles are the locations for the Yongquan acupoints of the kidney channels, which help to cure the deficiency syndrome of the kidneys and physical weakness. Modern medical research also affirms that washing the feet in warm water is a good stimulant for nerve endings, improves the memory, and relaxes the feet and brains.

Apart from using warm water, medicinal liquids can also be used to wash the feet to prevent and treat many senile diseases. Following are descriptions of some methods:

Heel pain: Tougucao (herb of tuberculate speranskia), Xungufeng (herb of woolly dutchmanspipe) and Laoguancao (heronbill), 30 g each; Huanghao (dried sweet wormwood) 20 g, Duhuo (pubescent angelica root) 15 g, Ruxiang (frankincense), Moyao (myrrh) and Xuejie (dragon's blood), 10 g each. Decoct them with water and wash the feet in the warm liquid, twice a day.

Ankle arthritis: Use the same prescription and the same method as for heel pain.

Foot injuries from falls, fractures, contusions and strains: Sumu (sappan wood), Zirantong (pyrite), 30 g each; peach kernel, Honghua (safflower), Tuyuan (ground beetles), Xuejie (dragon's blood), Ruxiang (frankincense), Moyao (myrrh), 12 g each. Decoct them with water, and wash the feet while it is warm, 2-3 times a day.

Vasculitis: Leech and earthworm, 30 g each; Chuanriuxi (cyathula root), Fuzi (prepared aconite lateral root), Guizhi (cassia twig), Gancao (liquorice root), 15 g each; Tuyuan (grownd beetles), peach kernel, Sumu (sappan wood), Honghua (safflower), Xuejie (dragon's blood), Ruxiang (frankincense), Moyao (myrrh), 10 g each. Decoct with water for 20 minutes. Decoct the dregs with water for another 60 minutes. Pour the liquids of the two decoctions together into a wooden tub and put the shanks and feet into the warm liquid.

Foot ulcers: Honeysuckle flowers, Lianqiao (forsythia fruit), Xiakucao (selfheal spike), Pugongying (dandelion), and Zihuadiding (violet), 30 g each; Danpi (root bark of tree peony), Huanglian (goldthread rhizome), Cangzhu (atractylodes rhizome), 10 g each. Decoct them with water and wash the injured foot or feet when the liquid is raised to 40 degrees Centigrade.

Beriberi: Use 100 g black plum to decoct with water. Wash the feet when the liquid cools, and then dry the feet with a clean towel, 1-3 times a day. Rubber-soled shoes or plastic shoes should not be used during the period of treatment and after the disease is cured. Cotton cloth shoes are recommended. The inside of the shoes should be kept clean and dry.

Red, itchy and sore eyes: Chrysanthemum flowers 60 g. Decoct with water and wash feet in the liquid, 1-3 times a day.

Hypertension: Xiakucao (selfheal spike), Gouteng (uncaria stem with hooks), mulberry leaf and chrysanthemum flower, 30 g each. Decoct with water and wash feet in the liquid. Once or twice a day, 10-15 minutes each time.

Dizziness: Use the same prescription and method as for hypertension.

Toothache due to wind-fire: Digupi (wolfberry bark) and gypsum, 60 g each; chrysanthemum 30 g, Fangfeng (saposhnikovia root) 15 g, tree peony bark 10 g. Decoct them with water and wash feet in the decoction 2-3 times a day, 5-10 minutes each time. Avoid pungent and greasy foods and eat less, especially at supper.

Frostbite: Guizhi (cassia twig), Fuzi (prepared aconite lateral root) and dried ginger, 15 g each. Decoct with water and wash feet while the decoction is warm, 2-3 times a day, 10-15 minutes each time.

Stubborn apathetic spasm of knees and ankles: Decoct chicken feathers 200 g with water, pour the decoction into a wooden tub, and put the feet and legs in decoction so that the affected parts with pathological changes are submerged in the liquid at a moderate temperature (around 50 degrees Centigrade). Be sure not to scald the skin.

Chapter Five

Sports and Leisure

For good health and a long life, middle-aged and older people should make their life as rich and colorful as possible. A peaceful and cozy environment, an optimistic and humorous temperament, and varied and broad interests make life happy and easy. This is very important for the health of body and mind.

1. A rich and colorful life

How do you make life rich and colorful? There are many ways. Cultural, sports and entertainment activities can be good for health, such as watching sports competitions, plays and dances, and listening to music. In traditional Chinese folk therapies, there is a therapy using the five notes of the ancient five-tone scale to treat diseases, because the five notes with rhyme can affect the five internal organs. In his *Records of the Historian*, Sima Qian mentioned about using music to excite the *qi* and blood. Modern science also confirms that beautiful musical melodies can relax a tense nervous system and produce a sedative and analgesic effect. It can also affect the functioning of the internal system. Music also helps regulate the secretion and flow of the blood and excite the mood and spirit of people.

Likewise, practicing calligraphy and painting, cultivating flowers and plants, and playing chess and cards are all activities beneficial to health.

In the following pages we will give special consideration to walking, running, kite-flying, touring and recuperation. These activities help cultivate the proper temperament for preserving good health and prolonging life.

2. Walking and running

(1) Walking

A Chinese proverb says: "If you wish to live to the age of 99, please walk 100 steps after each meal." Walking has been a good way of keeping healthy since ancient times.

Taking a walk after meals helps improve the secretion and peristalsis of the intestinal passages, shortens the time it take for food to enter the small intestine, promotes the digestion and absorption of food, and prevents stomach and intestinal disorders.

Walking is most beneficial for middle-aged and elderly people, and is the easiest and simplest form of physical exercise. It is also good for desk-bound workers and the physically weak and ill. If one walks in nature with fresh air, this benefits all systems of the human body, especially the muscles, joints, heart, and respiratory and nervous systems. Why?

An old saying goes: "The legs stiffen before a man becomes old." Nimble legs and feet are vital, and rhythmical walking is a good exercise for the muscles. While walking, keep the back straight and the arms swinging. By strengthening the activities of the muscles and joints of the legs you can prevent the stiffening and atrophy of the muscles and keep the joints nimble. The relaxation and contraction of the leg muscles while walking helps force the blood in the leg to flow back quickly to the heart. This is very good for stimulating blood circulation throughout the body.

Walking helps improve the functioning of the heart, promote the blood circulation of the coronary artery, and reduce both blood sugar and blood pressure. The contraction of the cardiac muscle quickens when you walk, enabling the heart to increase the blood supply and accelerate the blood flow. Rhythmical walking helps the body vibrate at a moderate and low frequency, which helps to temper the smooth muscles of the blood vessels, raising their tension. This helps prevent arteriosclerosis and diseases of the cerebral and cardiac blood vessels.

Walking is also good for the respiratory system. When you walk, you accelerate and deepen your breathing smoothly and rhythmically, and strengthen the movement of the diaphragmatic muscles to meet the demand for oxygen during muscular movement, thus enlarging the vital capacity, and improving the function of the respiratory system.

For sedentary workers, light and rhythmical walking helps alleviate nerve and muscle tension, increase the blood flow to the brain, and replenish nerve cells with more nutriments, thus alleviating cerebrum fatigue and calming the nervous system.

Walking also helps raise the body's metabolism rate and increase energy consumption. Moderate walking consumes 200 Calories an hour. If the pace is accelerated, this increases to 300-360 Calories. It is estimated that 0.45 kilograms of fat is lost for every 3,500 Calories burned. In other words, by walking for half an hour every day, all else being equal, 0.67 kilograms of fat will be gone in a month. Therefore, if a fat elderly man perseveres in walking every day, he will be able to reduce his weight and restore his health.

Practice has shown that walking is the best exercise for middle-aged and older people who are physically weak or suffer from heart trouble, hypertension, or obesity.

Walking as a form of physical exercise has its own requirements. The best place for walking is by a lake or a river, with woods, fresh air, a quiet environment, and a flat path. Or through park where the green color helps calm the nerves, lightens the burden on the heart and blood vessels, and regulates the air supply. Flowers in the park release many aromas that help to regulate the nerve center and kill germs and viruses.

Attention should also be paid to the clothes worn when walking. Don't wear too much clothing (be sure to keep the body warm in winter), and your shoes and socks should be light and well-fitted.

Attention should also be paid to your walking posture. Generally, keep the body straight, head up, chest out, eyes front and abdomen slightly withdrawn. The muscles of the buttocks should be tight, and the arms relax and swing naturally. The walking tempo should be even. Be sure not to walk quickly at one time and slowly at others.

Here, we would like to describe a walking method recorded in the *Illustrated Internal Qigong Exercise* a traditional physical exercise. It says: "Walking 100 steps with both hands massaging the abdomen helps dissolve the undigested food." That is to say, use both hands to massage the abdomen gently while walking to prevent and cure indigestion and chronic gastric and intestinal diseases.

(2)Running

Running as a physical exercise is becoming very popular. Some even regard running as the "perfect exercise."

What are the benefits of running?

First, running helps protect the heart. Older people often suffer from heart disease and deficiency of blood because their coronary arteries are blocked, which can lead to angina pectoris and myocardial infarction. Running helps the coronary artery maintain good blood circulation. Generally, running can prevent the coronary artery from shrinking or narrowing with age because of the blood supply and cardiac muscle stimulation and thereby help prevent coronary disease.

Secondly, running helps accelerate the circulation of blood throughout the body, adjust blood distribution, and remove the extravasated blood. Because a large muscle group contracts and relaxes alternately while running, it forces the blood in the veins to flow back, thus decreasing the extravasated blood in the leg veins and the pelvic cavity to prevent venous thrombosis.

Third, running helps metabolize fats, and prevent the excessive accumulation of fats in the blood to prevent high blood lipid diseases.

Fourth, running helps adjust the excitation and inhibition of the cerebral cortex, improve the function of the nervous system, relieve cerebrum fatigue and prevent neurasthenia.

Running is also a good way to combat obesity because it helps promote metabolism, consumes a large amount of energy and reduces the accumulation of fats to control weight.

Generally, middle-aged people are advised to do long-distance slow running while the older people should practise relaxed slow running. The running tempo depends on individual physique. The maximum load intensity should not exceed the rhythm of the heart at 120 beats per minute, and breathing should be moderate. While running, one should breathe deeply, long, gently, slowly and rhythmically. Use abdominal breathing as much as possible, that is, expand the belly when inhaling and empty the belly when exhaling. The strides should be light and the muscles relaxed, with the arms swinging naturally. The physical exertion should be properly controlled. Generally, running for 20 or 30 minutes everyday is best. At the start, one should run five to six times a week, or every other day. However, one must persevere in running before benefiting from it.

3. Kite-flying

China is the homeland of kites, and the Chinese people have been flying them for more than 2,000 years. The invention of kite-flying is regarded as a creation in imitation of the flight of birds. The inventor is said to be the legendary carpenter Lu Ban of the Spring and Autumn and Warring States periods. The legend says that he "cut the bamboo into a bird, made a kite and flew it for three days on end."

Kite-flying is not only an interesting pastime, but also can be an activity for improving physical fitness. Ancient Chinese physicians believed that "looking up with the mouth open while flying a kite helps to expel the internal heat," and that "flying a kite is the best way to improve eyesight."

Today, kite-flying is popular around the world. International kite-flying festivals are held in China every year and attract enthusiasts and master fliers from both at home and abroad. It has also come to be recognized by more and more people as a form of physical exercise.

Be sure not to fly a kite in bad weather, for example, on windy, rainy or snowy days. And fly kites far from power lines, high-tension cables in particular, to avoid danger. Do not fly a kite if you suffer from a disease which might attack suddenly. Nor should people suffering from serious coronary heart disease or angina pectoris do it.

Who are the best suited for the kite-flying therapy?

First, sufferers of hypertension and neurasthenia. When flying a kite, one has an ease of mind and a happy mood, thus relaxing the cerebral cortex and cerebral blood vessels. So it has a curing effect for hypertension and neurasthenia.

Second, people with dizziness, myopia and weak optic nerve.

When flying a kite, one looks up into the sky as far as he can, thus relieving the strain of the muscles around the eyes. This also helps cure dizziness and weak optic nerve.

Third, people with overaccumulated internal heat. Flying a kite in the fields with bright sunshine and fresh air helps to promote the circulation of blood and clear away the heat.

Besides, all sufferers of chronic diseases whose conditions are not serious can take kite-flying as a therapy to improve their physique and promote recovery.

Chapter Six

Proper Balance Between Work and Rest

There should be a proper balance between work and rest. This applies to both physical and mental work.

Work and rest are relative, not absolute, and there is no hard and fast line between them. Physical workers should read books or newspapers after work, and this is rest for them, just as the mental workers should engage in physical activities after work (as a way of relaxing). And this is rest for them. Everyone can benefit by physical exercise and recreation such as playing ball games or chess, singing songs or performing on the stage.

To keep in good health, work and recreation are both necessary to strike a proper balance. Either one in excess can be harmful to your health.

1. Work is good for health

An old saying goes: "The more you use your brains, the cleverer you become. The more you practise physical exercise, the stronger you are. Frequent use of the brains helps you look younger." All tissues and organs of the body "evolve when in use and degenerate when not in use." The more often they are used, the more developed they become. If they are not used, they quickly atrophy and becomes feeble. Although the cerebrum atrophies gradually at the beginning of middle age, this process can be slowed if it is constantly used. If the cerebrum, the high center of thought, does not atrophy, the physiological functions of all tissues and organs of the body can be maintained harmoniously and normally, thus slowing down the process of decline. Both in ancient times and today, many mental workers lived long lives. As already described in this book, Sun Simiao of the Tang Dynasty lived to 101 years, Zhen Quan 103 years, Qi Baishi, a famous modern painter, 97 years, and Ma Yinchu, a population theoretician, more than 100 years.

As physical strength gradually becomes weaker in middle age, work intensity should also be reduced. However, you should never stop working or being active. The less you work and move about, the more quickly your physical strength drops and the functions of the tissues and organs decline. Therefore, middle-aged and older people should be sure to do some physical work or exercise. This helps you not only limber up the muscles and bones, invigorate the circulation of blood and vital energy, and strengthen the function of the heart and metabolism, but also molds your temperament and broadens your mind.

Middle-aged and older people should never think that because they are aging, they should no longer be active, both physically and mentally. To think this way is to lose your vitality and grow old even more quickly. Remain active. Only in this way can the cerebral blood vessels maintain a state of diastole and the cells of the cerebrum be well preserved, thus slowing down the decline of the cerebrum and all tissues and organs of the body. Only in this way can you keep your spirit young and prolong your life.

2. Overwork is bad for health

Work is good for your health. Work here refers to the appropriate amount of work. Overwork or burdensome work can ruin your health; diseases caused by "physical overexertion" are called "work disease" in traditional Chinese medicine.

Questions and Answers says: "Protracted looking injures the blood, protracted lying injures the vital energy, protracted sitting injures the flesh, protracted standing injures the bones, and protracted walking injures the tendons. These are the injuries caused by five kinds of strain." It points out that protracted looking, lying, sitting, standing and walking can all injure the body and cause internal lesion. *Zhuang Zi (The Book of Master Zhuang)* says: "Nonstop physical work causes illness, and endless use of the mind causes internal lesions."

Why does overwork injure the body? Traditional Chinese medicine holds that overexertion harasses the Yang *qi* (masculine energy), generates excessive Yang *qi* and turns it into internal heat, thus destroying the balance between the Yin *qi* and Yang *qi* and causing illness. Excessive fatigue not only affects health, but may also endanger life.

With age, physiological functions of the internal organs decline, and physical strength and energy drop. Therefore, older folks should be careful not to become too fatigued. You must understand that "only when you have a good rest, can you do your work well" and "to rest is to do the work still better." Rest is not only needed for health, but also for work. A great man once said: "Only people who take a good rest can work well."

3. Rest is good for health

Rest helps kill fatigue, enhance vigor, restore physical strength and raise work efficiency to maintain the normal functions of the tissues and organs of the body. Moreover, it helps improve immunity and increase resistance to illness.

Traditional Chinese medicine advocates positive rest. What is "positive rest"? Positive rest does not mean merely sitting in a chair or lying on the bed. It means striking a balance between mental and physical work and changing activities to make life rich, colorful and significant. For example, when a physical worker is tired after work, he can sit down to read books or other material and engage in studies to increase his knowledge, or play chess or cards, and this is positive rest for him. When a mental worker feels tired, he can go outdoors, grow flowers and vegetables, breed fish, plant trees, play ballgames, ride a horse, take a walk, dance or climb a mountain. All this is positive rest for him.

4. Excessive rest can be harmful

Traditional Chinese medicine regards all excessive acts whether resting, sitting, lying, joy or sorrow or sex as harmful.

Traditional Chinese medicine calls diseases caused by excessive rest "diseases of ease." "Diseases of ease" are frequently found clinically. High-ranking officials, lords, and wealthy people may easily suffer from such diseases, commonly known as "diseases of wealth." Because these people live a good life, love ease and hate work, they may suffer from the "diseases of ease." An old Chinese saying goes: "Life springs from sorrow and calamity, and death from ease and pleasure."

The disease of ease is also common among retired people.

Because this disease is often found after retirement, some people call it "retirement syndrome." "Retirement syndrome" is one of the "diseases of ease." Its manifestations are listlessness, loneliness, vexation, worry, depression, exhaustion, palpitations, sweating, a dull life and lack of interest. A person suffering from retirement syndrome finds himself sleeping all day long after meals, doing nothing, and without objectives.

"Retirement syndrome" may last as long as three years. The time may be longer for some people and shorter for others. Some never recover from the syndrome.

Retirement is a common problem for everyone. If the problem is not well handled, one may fall into the "retirement syndrome." How can this be prevented? In plain words, avoid "excessive ease." It is essential to take a correct attitude toward life and set some goals for your remaining years. To make life rich and colorful, take part in more social activities on the basis of your interests, and have chats with friends to enrich knowledge and joy. In short, do not regard retirement as the end of life, but only one of life's milestones.

Chapter Seven

Health and Sex

Sex for health is a method of improving health through sexual activity. Ancient Chinese physicians attached great importance to the role of sex in health preservation. Despite the asceticism advocated by Buddhism and the Taoist idea of "less desire," the art of health preservation through sex has been passed down from generation.

1. Sex and health

Record of Rites says: "Food, drink, and man and woman are the major desires of a human being." Man and woman here means sexual acts between a man and a woman. In other words, food, drink and sex are essentials of human life. It regards sex as indispensable as food and drink and discusses the place of sex in maintaining health. Men and women marry and they must have a sex life, otherwise, they will fall ill. Sun Simiao, a great physician of the Tang Dynasty, believed that sex is valuable and essential to health. In his *The Thousand Golden Formulae* he says: "A man must have a woman, and a woman must have a man. If he has no woman, he thinks wild, if he thinks wild, it injures his mind, and if it injures the mind, it injures his health."

Even men at or over the age of 60 should have a moderate sex life. Sun says in the book that a strong man over 60 can have sex once a month, and if he is very strong physically, he can have sex any time he has the desire. Do not suppress it, he points out, and says that the older people should not have sex as frequently as the young, but they should not totally stop or suppress it.

When they mature sexually, men and women have sexual desires. This is a natural instinct of human beings. If a person reaches the proper age without getting married, or is divorced without remarriage, and cannot have their sexual desires gratified, they may easily become lovesick. Its manifestations are an unstable mood, irritability, unquiet sleep, lack of appetite, a sallow look, thinness and dejection. A man may have nocturnal emissions while a woman may dream of intercourse, menstrual disorder or endocrinopathy. Some people even become mentally deranged because of a broken marriage or love affair, the loss of a spouse, or the failure to have intercourse with the opposite sex.

Regular and harmonious sex helps make married couples physically and mentally healthy, deepen their love, and increase family harmony, thus benefiting health and long life. Many investigations have shown that lack of regular and harmonious sex is an important cause of worsening family relations and broken marriages. Worsening family relations or broken marriages, in turn, give rise to a bad state of mind, not only affecting health, but also shortening life.

What harm does overindulging in sex do to health?

Appropriate and moderate sex not only is harmless, but is beneficial to health. However, excessive sex may harm one's health.

In traditional Chinese medicine, the term "sexual strain" refers to internal lesions caused by excessive sex. According to Chinese medicine, among the internal lesions caused by overexertion, "sexual strain" is the most serious one. Therefore, physicians in all dynasties took great pains to warn people against a greed for sex and against excessive sex.

Modern research indicates that sex has a major affect on the human body. Apart from the discharge of semen by men, both men and women will discharge a large amount of fluid and various hormones from the sex glands. These substances are produced within the body at a high cost, and greatly affect health. Excessive sex brings great losses of these precious substances, thus harming both men and women, but even more harm to men. The fluid discharge by men is a mixture of semen, prostate fluid and sex hormone, products of the testis. Excessive sex and excessive ejaculation naturally increases the burden on the testis and accelerates their atrophy. Atrophy of the testis and the decreasing secretion of the sex hormone, in turn, accelerates the decline of the body. This is why excessive sex leads to early decline and early death. It also explains why the theory of "excessive sex injuring the kidneys" in traditional Chinese medicine is scientifically founded. The short life of many emperors in all dynasties was largely caused by their unrestrained sexual activity.

To sum up, both the prohibition of sex and its excess are harmful to health. Only proper and moderate sex is good for health and beneficial for a long life.

2. Sex for middle-aged and older people

What is moderate sex? The physical strength and energy of most middle-aged and older people gradually become weak, and their sexual function also weakens. They should reduce the number of times for sex. Traditional Chinese medicine attaches great importance to the effect of "kidney semen," and believes that excessive sex does damage to the kidney semen and injures the body. Therefore, specialists in all dynasties have exhorted the people to control their sexual activity. It is appropriate for people in their forties to have sex once a week, people in their fifties once every two weeks, and people in their sixties once a month. People in poor health should have even less sex. Sick people should stop sex for the time being and restore sex after recovery. People with chronic diseases such as hypertension, coronary heart disease, diabetes and senile chronic bronchitis should, apart from reducing sex, not be too excited or stimulated so as to avoid accidents. When sexual activity reaches a climax of excitement, the heartbeat speeds up to 120-180 per minute and the rhythm of breathing also rise to 60 per minute, and blood pressure rises. Sexual intercourse is not a very strenuous activity, but it presents a threat to those sufferering from hypertension and coronary heart disease. An old Chinese saying goes: "The affair in the bedroom can either kill people or give births. If used properly, it helps to improve health. If not used properly, it can cause death immediately."

3. Sex hygiene

Middle-aged and older people should not have sex when they feel tired, and old people who cannot manage their own day-to-day life should avoid sex altogether. If they are completely exhausted or suffer from serious diseases, sex can be very harmful.

People should avoid sex after meals, drinking (after banquets in particular) or bathing, or when they are very nervous. Sun Simiao said: "There should be never intercourse after a bath, when tired after travel, after meals or when drunk, in great joy or in great sorrow, when man or woman have a fever (flu and typhoid), or when a woman has menses or has just given birth."

If you are attacked by wind after sex, this may easily cause facial paralysis and even cerebral stroke. If you sleep in the open air after sex, you may easily suffer from rheumatic arthritis, aching muscles and bones, and spasms. Do not eat cold food or drink cold water or take a cold bath, because this may cause violent abdominal pains, the shrinkage of the vulva, and even death.

Chapter Eight

Learn to Do Exercises

There are many traditional exercises popular among the Chinese people that are simple and easy to learn and practise.

1. "Sixteen should's for health preservation"

The "16 should's" are a traditional set of Chinese exercises for health preservation based on *qigong* which were widely practised as early as the Ming Dynasty.

The "16 should's for health preservation" refer to 16 points or aspects concerning health. According to classical records, the 16 points are as follows:

"The hair should be frequently combed, the face should be frequently rubbed, the eyes should be frequently exercised, the ears should be frequently flicked, the teeth should be frequently clicked, the tongue should frequently lick the palate, the saliva should be frequently swallowed, the stale air should be frequently exhaled, the abdomen should be frequently massaged, the anus should be frequently contracted, the limbs should be frequently shaken, the soles of the feet should be frequently rubbed, the skin should be frequently rubbed, the back should always be kept warm, the chest should always be well covered, and silence should be kept when having bowel movements or passing water."

Specifically, these exercises should be done as follows:

(1) The hair should be frequently combed: Bend all fingers and

use them as a comb. Comb the hair from the forehead to the back of the head, and do it repeatedly. Comb around 100 strokes each time. Do it gently and slowly. The result is even better if it is done in the morning. Because this stimulates and massages the acupoints on the head, it helps to kill pain, improve sight and reduce blood pressure.

(2) The face should be frequently rubbed: Rub the hands until they are warm then place them on your face, with the middle fingers on the sides of the nose. Start from the Yingxiang acupoints and rub gently upward to the forehead and then to both sides and cheeks. Rub this way 30 times, preferably in the morning. This helps refresh the head and reduce blood pressure. It also helps to reduce wrinkles.

(3) The eyes should be frequently exercised: In exercising the eyes, the eyeballs should be turned slowly from left to right 14 times, and then from right to left 14 times. Close the eyes tightly after the exercise and then open them suddenly. This helps improve your eyesight.

(4) The ears should be frequently flicked: First cover the ears with both palms, with the three fingers in the middle hitting the occiput gently 12 times. Then press the forefinger on the middle finger and then slip it down to snap the back of the head 12 times with clear cracking sounds. Do it after arising in the morning or when you feel tired. This helps cure tinnitus, dizziness and ear ailments. It also helps improve hearing and memory.

(5) The teeth should be frequently clicked: Close the mouth gently and tap the upper and lower teeth together lightly. First tap the molars 24 times and then tap the front teeth 24 times. This helps improve the teeth.

(6) The tongue should frequently lick the palate: Put the tip of the tongue against the upper palate or use the tip of the tongue to lick the upper palate so that Yin and Yang meet each other. When

licking, focus attention under the tongue, feeling that saliva comes out gradually.

(7) The saliva should be frequently swallowed: When the tongue licks the upper palate, a large amount of saliva comes out. Traditional Chinese medicine attaches great importance to saliva, calling it "golden fluid," a treasure of the human body. Swallow the saliva down slowly to irrigate the internal organs and moisten the limbs and hair, promote digestion and absorption, and improve the function of the intestines and stomach. When the mouth is full of saliva, bulge the cheeks, gargle 36 times and then swallow it slowly, preferably with gurgling sounds, using the mind to send it to Dantian below the navel.

(8) The stale air should be frequently exhaled: Hold the breath at the beginning to bulge the chest and abdomen. When you feel both the chest and abdomen filled with air, raise the head slightly and open the mouth slowly to exhale the stale air from the chest and abdomen. Repeat the exercise 5 to 7 times. It helps expel the accumulated stale air, open the chest to smooth the breathing, and stop asthma and pain.

(9) The abdomen should be frequently massaged: First rub the hands until they are warm, and then place them on the navel, with the left hand on top of the right hand for men, and the opposite for women. Move them around the navel with the palm clockwise from small circles to large circles 36 times, and then counterclockwise from large circles to small circles 36 times. This helps promote the peristalsis of the stomach and intestines, smooth the breathing, remove food stagnancy, improve the digestive and absorptive functions, and prevent and cure gastric and intestinal diseases.

(10) The anus should be frequently contracted: First draw in a full breath, and then contract the anus with force, and raise it together with the perineum. Pause for a moment, relax and let out the

air slowly. Repeat the exercise 5 to 7 times. This helps raise Yang *qi*, and prevent and cure haemorrhoids, prolapse of the anus, and anal fistula.

(11) The limbs should be frequently shaken: Clench both hands tightly, pivot on the waist and turn the shoulders from left to right as if turning a wheel 24 times, and then from right to left 24 times. Sit in a chair and first raise the left leg and extend it slowly forward, toes upward. When the leg is almost straight, kick the heel forward and downward with a moderate force. Then change to the right leg and do it the same way. Repeat the exercise 5 times. This helps stretch the limbs and joints, remove obstructions in meridians and collaterals, prevent and cure aching joints, and strengthen the legs.

(12) The soles should be frequently rubbed: Before going to bed, warm the hands by rubbing them after washing the feet, and then rub the Yongquan acupoints on the soles. Keep on circling slowly 50 to 100 times. This helps strengthen the kidneys, warm the feet, communicate between the heart and the kidneys, soothe the liver, and improve the eyesight.

(13) The skin should be frequently rubbed: Stroke and rub the skin all over the body. First rub the palms warm and then stroke and rub the skin in the following order: Start from the Baihui acupoint on the top of the head, and then rub the face, down the left and right shoulders and arms, chest, and abdomen to the ribs on both sides. Then rub the two sides of the waist, and finally the left and right legs. This helps promote the smooth circulation of blood and vital energy and polish the skin.

(14) and (15) Keep the back warm and the chest well covered all the time, and (16) keep silence while having a bowel movement and passing water: According to traditional Chinese medicine, the human body has two major channels and collateral: The Du channel that passes along the midline of the back and is the sea of the Yang

meridians, and the Ren channel that passes along the midline of the chest and abdomen and is the sea of the Yin meridians. So it is very important to protect the chest and back since they bear on the normal operation of the Du and Ren channels. Look up and keep the mouth tightly shut while having a bowel movement and passing water in order to prevent the discharge of the vital substances.

These 16 "should's" for health preservation are quite scientifically founded, and have therefore been widely practised. When doing the exercises, concentrate the mind, keep quiet and calm, and move slowly and breathe naturally. You will benefit if you persevere step by step in an orderly way.

2. Lao Zi's brain exercises

Lao Zi was a thinker during the Spring and Autumn period (770-476 B.C.) in China, and the founder of Taoism. Legend has it that he worked out a set of exercises for invigorating the cerebral function. The following is a description of the set of exercises sorted out by people of later generations:

(1) Open the Yintang acupoint: Yintang is located at the midpoint between the eyebrows. Use the tips of the thumbs to turn-rub the temples several times and then use the cushion of the middle fingers to rub the Yintang acupoint 16 times. (Fig. 8-1)

(2) Rub the eyes: Rub the eye sockets and their surroundings 16 times simultaneously with the forefinger tips. (Fig. 8-2)

(3) Push the Dicang acupoints: Dicang are located about 1.5 cm from the corners of the mouth. When doing this exercise, open the mouth slightly and use the thumb tips to press and push Dicang 16 times. (Fig. 8-3)

(4) Point-press the Sibai acupoints: Sibai are located about 1.5 cm under both eye sockets. Use the forefinger tips to point-

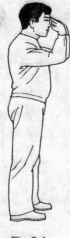

Fig. 8-1

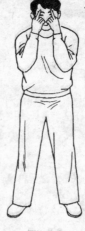

Fig. 8-2

press the Sibai from bottom upward 16 times. (Fig. 8-4)

(5) Rub the nose: Use the thenars of both hands to rub the nose 16 times. (Fig. 8-5)

(6) Rub the neck: Place both palms on both sides of the neck and rub the neck from above downward 16 times. (Fig. 8-6)

(7) Wash the face like a cat: Use both palms to rub the face 16 times. (Fig. 8-7)

(8) Comb the hair: Separate the fingers and rub the head from the forehead to the back of the head. Run the finger tips through the hair to massage the major tendons and blood vessels on the head. Comb in this way 16 times. (Fig. 8-8)

(9) Sound the celestial drum: Use both palms to cover the ears, with the thumbs and middle fingers joining together to snap the Fengchi acupoints below the occipital bone 16 times. (Fig. 8-9)

After finishing these 9 exercises, use both palms to press tight the ears for a moment, and then take them off with force. Repeat 3-

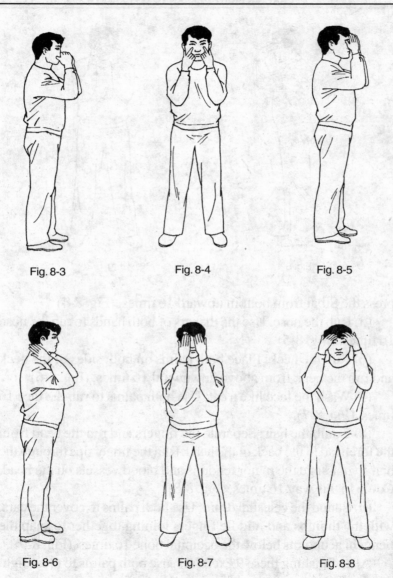

Fig. 8-3   Fig. 8-4   Fig. 8-5

Fig. 8-6   Fig. 8-7   Fig. 8-8

5 times, and the whole set is completed.

3. Hair-combing exercises

People in ancient China did some research on the relation between hair combing and health preservation, and wrote of their research results in books. For example, it is pointed out in one of such books: "Apart from food and exercise, there are two major points for health preservation: hair-combing and washing the feet."

Combing the hair frequently not only helps to dispel wind, remove heat and nourish the hair, but also benefits health in general. Of course, the combing the ancient people had in mind is not the same as that in modern life. Theirs was in fact a kind of massaging exercises using the hands instead of a comb. This kind of exercise has been handed down to the present day after generations of practice and modification.

The combing exercise is a method of massaging the head at seven acupoints. They are (Fig. 8-10):

(1) Zanzhu, located on the medial extremity of the eyebrows;

(2) Shenting, located at the midpoint on the borderline between the forehead and the hair;

(3) Qianding, located at the top of the front skull;

(4) Naohu, a major acupoint located in the depression at the rear of the skull;

(5) Erhou, located in the depression behind the ears;

(6) Egu, located at the bottom end of the ears;

(7) Tianmen, located at the bone of the top end of the ears.

The combing massage is done like this:

(1) First bend the fingers of both hands like rakes, with the thumbs on the Tianmen acupoints and the other fingers separated at equal distances, the little fingers just on the Zanzhu acupoints. This is the

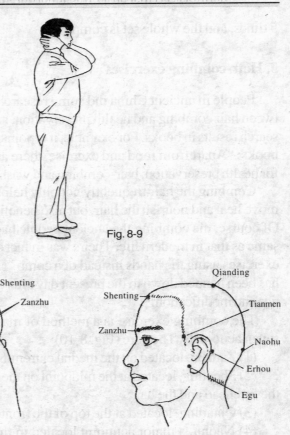

Fig. 8-9

Fig. 8-10

starting position.

(2) In starting the exercise, push the five fingers upward at the same time as if scratching an itch, with the little fingers as the center, passing across Shenting to Qianding. While pushing to the back of the head, use the forefingers to press Naohu. Then use the thumbs to press Erhou. Finally, turn the fingers to Egu and again to Tianmen

to make one circle. It takes about five seconds. After this exercise, the blood in all the vessels of the skull are invigorated.

Massaging these acupoints correctly this way not only helps invigorate the circulation of the blood in the vessels of the cortex of the head, but also improves the cerebral function and prevents dizziness. Perseverance in this exercise also helps promote the growth of new hair, make gray hair black and shining, facial skin tender, and remove spots on the face. Some people even grow new hair on their bald head.

This exercise should be done neither too fast nor too slow. Keep cheerful. The exercise should be repeated 30 times every morning and evening respectively. It takes about two and a half minutes and you can do it while lying, sitting, standing or walking.

4. Exercises for the sense organs

The mouth, nose, eyes and ears are sense organs. The traditional Chinese medicine holds that the sense organs are closely related to the internal organs. For example, the tongue is related to the heart, the eyes to the liver, the kidneys to the ears, the lungs to the nose, and the philtrum, or groove of upper lip. Therefore, the health of the sense organs have direct influence on the internal organs.

(1) Description of six traditional sets of exercises for the sense organs:

[1] Eye exercise:

Keep the head straight up, eyes closed, turning the eyeballs from left to right 9 times and then from right to left 9 times. Open the eyes and look obliquely upward 9 times and downward 9 times. Do the exercise repeatedly and frequently. It helps prevent the decline of eyesight in middle-aged and older people.

[2] Tongue exercise

Use the tongue to lick the upper jaw when inhaling, uttering the sound of "hush" silently in the mind, and pause for a moment. Keep on licking the upper jaw with the tongue, silently uttering the sound of "her." At this time, direct the air into the lower abdomen, drop the tip of the tongue slowly and exhale the air slowly, silently uttering the sound of "si." This exercise helps link the Du channel with the Ren channel, and generate semen and preserve bodily fluid. (The Du and Ren are two of the eight extra meridians. The former is the sea of the Yang meridians, which governs all Yang meridians. The latter is the sea of the Yin meridians, which directs all Yin meridians.)

[3] Ear exercise

Use the cushions of both thumbs to massage the back of the ears gently from below upward 49 times, and then place the tips of the little fingers into the ears and shake them 49 times. Pull them out abruptly. Use the middle fingers to press the ears and tragus, and close them 49 times.

This exercise has a curing effect for tinnitus and non-infected earaches.

[4] Renzhong exercise

Close the eyes, use the end of one thumb to repeatedly massage and press lightly on the Renzhong acupoint (the midpoint in the groove of the upper lip). This exercise helps treat Meniere's disease and temporary absentmindedness.

[5] Yingxiang exercise

Use the cushions of both middle fingers to rub the Yingxiang acupoints on both sides of the nose back and forth until they become warm. Use the internal energy of the fingers to nourish Yingxiang. (Yingxiang are located on both sides of the nose, in the nasolabial groove, beside the midpoint of the lateral border of the ala nasi.)

This exercise helps prevent and cure frostbite of the nose and acne.

[6] Teeth exercise

The traditional teeth clicking exercise include teeth clicking, saliva mixing, rinsing with saliva, and bulging. It is done this way:

After getting up in the morning or before going to bed in the evening, click the molars first and then the front teeth, and then the right and left canine teeth; click them separately. Do it this way because the teeth are not on the same level, and it is impossible to click them all at the same time.

After clicking the teeth each time, use the tongue to stir around the bases of the teeth along the gums and the membrane of the cheeks. When a lot of saliva is secreted, keep it in the mouth and rinse the teeth several times. Then swallow the saliva down slowly. Traditional Chinese medicine incorporates the idea that saliva is a bodily fluid which should not be spat out.

Then use the tongue to massage the gums. This helps invigorate the smooth circulation of blood in the gums. Clench the teeth tightly and keep bulging the cheeks. This will also produce a lot of saliva in the mouth, which should also be swallowed down slowly. These exercises take about 10 minutes. There is no limit to how many times the exercises should be done, but you must repeat the exercises at least 40 to 50 times. There is no limit even if you want to do it several hundred times.

By the way, we would like to introduce another teeth-strengthening method. Close the eyes, hold the breath and clench the teeth when you pass water. This is called "close the celestial gate." It also helps strengthen the teeth. Many old people use this method to protect their teeth. Why are the teeth strengthened by clenching them? This is because when you clench the teeth, the base of the teeth is massaged, the blood flow is invigorated, and the teeth naturally become strong and firm. As the teeth are the first instrument for the nourishment of the body, strengthening the teeth all year round benefits the entire body. This is why perseverance in clicking the teeth helps to prolong life.

(2) Eye exercise

It has been a wide practice since ancient times to use eye exercise and self-massage to protect eyesight. According to ancient records, the common methods used are as follows:

[1] Turn the eyeballs to the left and to the right 7 times respectively. Close the eyes tightly for a while and then open them suddenly.

[2] Use the hands to press the Xiao Xuezhong acupoints at the outer corners of the eyes 27 times.

[3] Use the backs of the thumbs to press Xiao Xuezhong 36 times respectively, and then press the corners of the eyes close to the nose 36 times.

Following is the description of a common set of eye exercises (Fig. 8-11)

[1] Knead the Tianying acupoints: Close the eyes, press and knead the upper sockets of both eyes under the eyebrows with the cushions of the thumbs.

[2] Push and press the Jingming acupoints: Use the left or right thumb and index finger to push and press the root of the nose, first press downward and then push upward.

[3] Rub the Sibai acupoints: First put the index fingers and middle fingers of both hands together on the two sides of the nose, with the thumbs supporting the depression of the lower jaw bone, the middle, ring and little fingers bent inward, and use the index fingers to rub and press the central part of the cheeks (a finger's space below the midpoint of the lower eye sockets).

[4] Press the temples and massage the eye sockets: Bend the four fingers inward, and use the cushions of the thumbs to press the temples, and the inner sides of the second sections of the forefingers

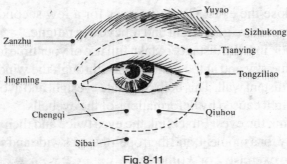

Fig. 8-11

to massage the eye sockets in a circle lightly, first the upper sockets, and then the lower sockets (that is, in the direction of inside up, outside up, outside down and inside down) so that all the acupoints on the eye sockets such as Zanzhu, Yuyao, Sizhukong and Tongziliao and Chengqi are pressed and massaged.

Do these exercises once or twice a day, and each of the massaging exercises 20 to 30 times. The location of the acupoints must be accurate, the movements must be gentle and slow until you get a sense of numbness and soreness.

(3) Sixteen-point eye exercises for eyesight protection

[1] Massage the face: Use one hand to massage the face, with movements looking like a cat washing its face. The massage should focus on the eyebrows and eyes. You do not have to do it too long. The massage is finished when the facial skin feels slightly warm. (Fig. 8-12)

[2] Rub the head: Use all five fingers of one hand or the fingers of both hands to rub the roots of the hair so that the head becomes clear and the eyes become bright. (Fig. 8-13)

[3] Beat the drum: Use all the fingers of both hands to beat the head, from the forehead to the back of the head. This has a good effect on the eyesight. (Fig. 8-14)

[4] Close the eyes: Close the eyes for a few seconds to one minute to preserve good sight and relieve eye fatigue.

[5] Look into the distance: Make full use of your time to look up into the blue sky and at the white clouds through the window or at spots on a distant wall. This helps regulate eyesight and avoid weakened eyesight caused by deformations of the eyeballs.

[6] Blink the eyes: First blink the eyes twice and then close the eyes tightly for a moment, and then open the eyes wide and suddenly. Repeat the exercise 2 or 3 times.

[7] Look around: Keep your head erect, with the eyeballs only slipping to left and right, and repeat the exercise several times.

[8] Glare like a tiger: Twist the neck to look backward 4 to 5 times, alternately on the left and right. This helps prevent and cure cervical vertebra disease as well as improve the eyesight. (Fig. 8-15)

[9] Stare: Open your eyes wide and look with close attention at a certain target inside or outside the room. The target should be at the same or slightly lower than eye level. Close the eyes for a while after staring and think of the visual image in your mind. Repeat the exercise 2 or 3 times. It helps improve both eyesight and memory.

[10] Turn the eyeballs: After waking up in the morning, first turn the eyeballs clockwise and counterclockwise 4 to 5 times respectively with the eyes closed, and then do it in the same way with the eyes open. In the evening, first turn the eyeballs with the eyes open, and then turn the eyeballs with the eyes closed.

[11] Iron the eyes: Rub your palms together forcefully until the palms become warm. Then use the palms to iron the eyes and press the eyes lightly several times. (Fig. 8-16)

[12] Point-pressing: Use the knuckles of the forefingers or thumbs to press a few times the acupoints on and around the eyes and eyebrows (Fig. 8-11), but only one or two pairs by rotation each

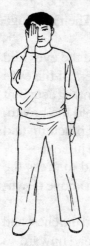

Fig. 8-12

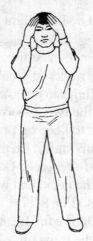

Fig. 8-13

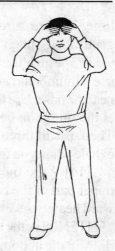

Fig. 8-14

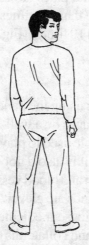

Fig. 8-15

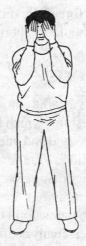

Fig. 8-16

time. The pressure should be from light to heavy. Then massage gently for a while.

[13] Pinch the eye corners near the nose: Close the eyes and use a thumb and a middle finger to pinch the corners of the eyes near the nose. Use the forefinger to point-press the Yintang acupoint at the midpoint between the two eyebrows and hold the breath. Then use all three fingers to keep on pressing and pinching and exhale when you feel slightly stuffy. Do this exercise just once.

[14] Wipe the back of the neck: Use one hand to press the upper part of the back of the neck, and wipe it from above downward heavily several times. (Fig. 8-17)

[15] Relax the spine: Draw a full breath to expand the chest and draw in the abdomen. At the same time, raise the head upward so as to pull the spinal column upward as much as possible, and then exhale and return to the original position.

[16] Rub the ribs: Use the bases of the palms to rub the ribs slowly but forcefully on both sides more than 10 times, and then shrug the shoulders alternately more than 10 times. (Fig. 8-18)

5. Finger exercises

There is a game among Chinese folks using the hands to make different gestures which form shadow images on a wall. These images can be vivid and interesting and people used to play this game to tease children, but few of them know it is also a good exercise with an invigorating effect on the cerebrum and blood vessels. There is a common saying: "People with deft hands are clever."

From the viewpoint of traditional Chinese medicine, there are on the fingers many acupoints, channels and collaterals that have a close bearing on health. Proper stimulation of these points, channels and collaterals can help maintain good health and relieve illness.

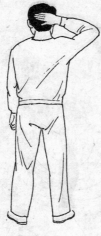

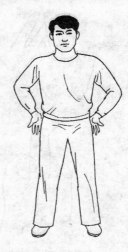

Fig. 8-17   Fig. 8-18

In the evenings, find some time to play this game with your children. It not only benefits your health and the health of your children, but also makes the family atmosphere more cheerful and stimulates children's imaginations. You can shoot three birds with one stone.

Following are descriptions of some simple games, from which you can also create many more interesting patterns:

[1] Shrimp: Cross the little and ring fingers and use the forefingers to touch the tip of the crossed ring fingers. Put the middle fingers together and straighten them out, and spread or bend the thumb gently. The shadow image reflected on the wall is now a lively shrimp. (Fig. 8-19)

[2] Horse: Put the hands together tightly. Straighten the little fingers and cross the ring and middle fingers. Bend the thumbs opposite each other to form a horse head on the wall. (Fig. 8-20)

[3] Dog: Use the four fingers of the right hand to cover the outer side of the left forefinger. Put the forefinger and middle fingers of the

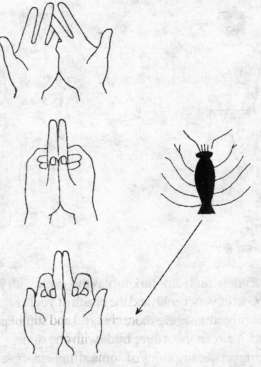

Fig. 8-19

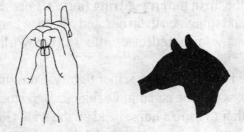

Fig. 8-20

left hand together, and the ring and little fingers together to open and close them. This now appears as a fierce dog when reflected on the wall. (Fig. 8-21)

[4] Rabbit: Put the hands together back to back, with the little fingers and forefingers hooked together. The middle and ring fingers can now move freely. The two fingers above look like the ears while the fingers below look like the rabbit's legs, and the strightened thumb of the lower hand looks like the tail. (Fig. 8-22)

[5] Owl: Cross the little and ring fingers and use the forefingers to keep the ring fingers under. Put the middle fingers together and bend them forward. Then let the tips of the thumbs and forefingers touch each other to form an owl head. (Fig. 8-23)

6. Finger-bending exercises

Traditional Chinese medicine holds that the meridian system of the human body consists mainly of three Yin meridians of the hand, three Yin meridians of the foot, three Yang meridians of the hand and three Yang meridians of the foot. These 12 meridians are the main channels and collaterals for the flow of blood and *qi* (vital energy), and form the main body of the meridian system. This system plays an important role in the physiological functions and pathological changes of the body, and gives guidance to medical treatment.

The 12 meridians are: The lung meridian of hand Taiyang, the large intestine meridian of hand Yangming, the stomach meridian of foot Yangming, the spleen meridian of foot Taiyin, the heart meridian of hand Shaoyin, the small intestine meridian of hand Taiyin, the bladder meridian of foot Taiyang, the kidney meridian of foot Shaoyin, the pericardium meridian of hand Jueyin, the triple energizer meridian of hand Shaoyang, the gallbaldder meridian of foot Shaoyang, and the liver meridian of foot Jueyin.

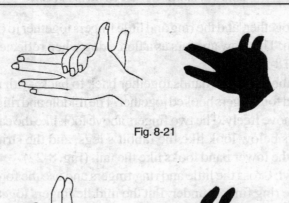

Fig. 8-21

Fig. 8-22

The main directions of their passage are: The three Yin meridians of the hand pass from the chest to the hand, the three Yang meridians of the hand pass from the hand to the head, the three Yin meridians of the foot pass from the foot to the abdomen and the three Yang meridians of the foot pass from the head to the feet. In addition, there are many other complicated channels and collaterals.

The finger-bending exercises are precisely based on the theory of the 12 meridians and are effective in adjusting the cycle of the meridians. It is particularly good for regulating the functions of the heart and the cerebrum and helps prevent and cure cardiovascular and cerebral diseases.

They are done in this way:

Starting position: Sit erect on a chair (with the back away from

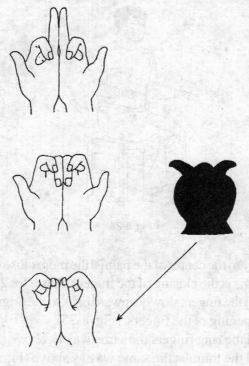

Fig. 8-23

the back of the chair), back straight, chest out and belly in, shoulders relaxed, arms down, and with some empty space under the armpits, enough to hold an egg. Bend the elbows, hands stretching level and palms down in the shape of a tile, tongue licking the upper palate, molars tightly clenched and eyes slightly closed. (Fig. 8-24)

The order of finger-bending is: 2, 4, 1, 5, 3, that is, the forefinger, ring finger, thumb, little finger and middle finger.

To bend the fingers is to close and open the fingers.

[1] Bend the forefingers: Bend the forefingers slowly downward

123

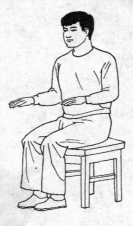

Fig. 8-24

and gradually to the center of the palms, the more close to the center, the better. This is the closing of the fingers. Pause for 20 seconds to 1 minute. Lift the fingers slowly upward back to the original position. This is the opening of the fingers. (Fig. 8-25)

[2] Bend the ring fingers the same way as above (Fig. 8-26)

[3] Bend the thumbs the same way as above (Fig. 8-27)

[4] Bend the little fingers the same way as above (Fig. 8-28)

[5] Bend the middle fingers the same way as above (Fig. 8-29)

When bending the fingers it is most desirable to bend the corresponding toes at the same time. It is relatively difficult to bend the toes one by one, but still try to do it in the order 2, 4, 1, 5, 3. It is more effective if the mind is used to guide the bending. It is said that the most skillful people can bend their toes one by one with ease.

After bending the five fingers, raise the palms upward slowly, and use the nose to breathe deeply (Fig. 8-30). When the hands are raised to chest level, press the up-turned palms slowly downward, and at the same time use the mouth to breathe out. (Fig. 8-31)

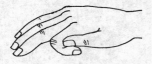

Fig. 8-25

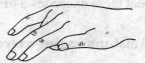

Fig. 8-26

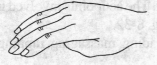

Fig. 8-27

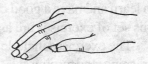

Fig. 8-28

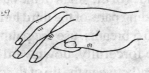

Fig. 8-29

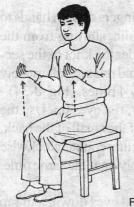

Fig. 8-30

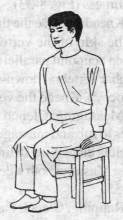

Fig. 8-31

125

Repeat these exercises 3 to 5 times.

7. Waist-massaging exercises

Waist-massaging exercises are a good set of exercises for maintaining a healthy waist. It also serves as physical therapy for treating functional diseases of the waist. These exercises are simple and easy to learn and have a good curative effect. The acupoints involved in this set of exercises are as shown in Fig. 8-32.

The exercises include rubbing, kneading, massaging, rapping, grasping, and turning.

[1] Rubbing: Sit up straight, feet apart to shoulder width, and rub the palms several dozen times. When they become warm, press them tightly on both sides of the small of the back (in the depression 10 cm from the protruding parts of the third lumbar vertebra). After pausing for about 3 to 5 breaths, use the palms to rub the sides of the lumbar vertebrae forcefully, downward to the Changqiang acupoint of the coccyx (between the tip of the coccyx and the anus, and upward to as far as the bent arms can reach). Repeat the exercise 36 timess (Fig. 8-33)

[2] Kneading: Use the thumbs and forefingers of both hands to knead the skin of the vertebrae in the middle, starting from the Mingmen acupoint parallel to the navel (under the knot of the second lumbar vertebra) downward, kneading and relaxing alternately to the coccyx. Knead the vertebrae this way 4 times. (Fig. 8-34)

[3] Massaging: Clench the fists loosely, fist eyes up. Use the knuckles to rub and massage the two sides of the small of the back, first circling clockwise 18 times and then circling counterclockwise 18 times. Massage both sides either separately or at the same time. (Fig. 8-35)

[4] Rapping: Clench the fists loosely, fist eyes down, and rap

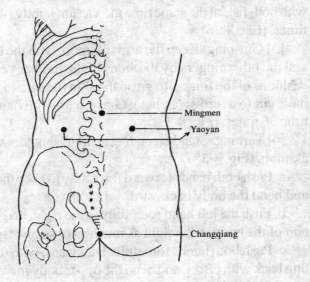

Mingmen

Yaoyan

Changqiang

Fig. 8-32

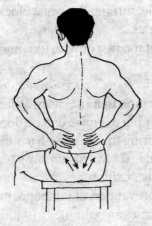

Fig. 8-33

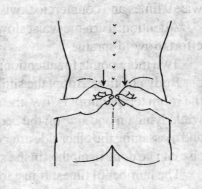

Fig. 8-34

with both fists at the same time the sacrum lightly (without pain) 36 times. (Fig. 8-36)

[5] Grasping: Keep the arms akimbo, with the thumbs in front and the other fingers by the sides of the lumbar vertebra. Use the cushions of the fingers to grasp the skin (be sure to have the finger nails cut to avoid scratches). Grasp with both hands at the same time 36 times. (Fig. 8-37)

[6] Turning: Stand erect, feet apart to shoulder width and arms akimbo. (Fig. 8-38)

a. Push both hands forward forcefully to keep the abdomen out, and bend the body backward.

b. Push the left hand forcefully to the right, and bend the upper part of the body to the right as much as possible.

c. Push both hands forcefully backward, with the buttocks sitting back with effort, and bend the upper body forward as much as possible.

d. Push the right hand forcefully to the left, and bend the upper body to the left as much as possible.

The four movements form one cycle, turning the waist clockwise 9 times and counterclockwise 9 times.

Attention: Turn the waist slowly, not too fast or with too much effort to avoid sprain.

Two more points for attention:

Body position: Adopt the sitting position in most cases. When the room temperature is low, the massaging exercise can be done while lying on one side on the bed, covering the body with a quilt, and massaging the other side after one side. The waist-turning exercise can be done in clothes in the standing position.

The number of times: If just for the prevention of lumbago, the number of times for massage in each exercise can be limited to within 36 times. If for medical treatment, the number of times can be in-

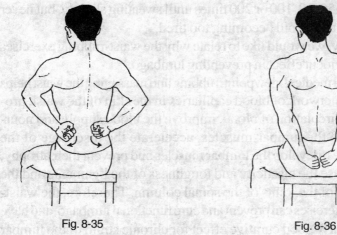

Fig. 8-35

Fig. 8-36

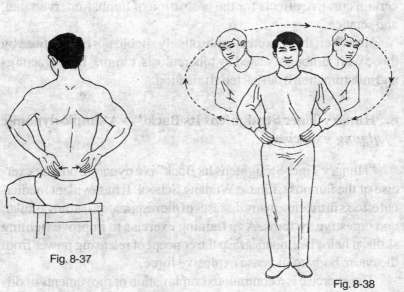

Fig. 8-37

Fig. 8-38

creased to 50, 60, 100 or 200 times until sweating slightly, but never overdo it, and avoid becoming too tired.

Finally, we would like to relate why the waist-rubbing exercises have an evident effect in preventing lumbago.

From a medical viewpoint, rubbing and massaging the waist helps dilate the network of blood capillaries in the skin of the waist, promote the circulation of blood, improve the blood supply and nourishment to the lumbar muscles, accelerate the discharge of the metabolites, develop the lumbar muscles and prevent their atrophy, and increase the elasticity and toughness of the ligaments and the flexibility of the joints of the spinal column. Therefore, the waist-rubbing exercises can prevent and cure functional lumbago, and have a particularly good curative effect for chronic strain of the lumbar muscles, acute lumbar sprains, and common lumbago. It also has certain curative effects for the protrusion of lumbar intervertabal, and sciatica.

However, these exercises absolutely should not be practised by those with lumbago caused by tuberculosis, tumors, bone fractures and inflammation from bacterial infection.

8. "Hungry Tiger Straightens Its Back"— A simple dynamic *qigong* exercise

"Hungry Tiger Straightens Its Back" is a dynamic boxing exercise of the famous Chinese Wudang School. It has evident medicinal effects in treating many diseases of the respiratory, cardiovascular, and digestive systems. As a training exercise to improve fighting skills, it helps beginners grasp the concept of releasing power from the entire body to increase explosive force.

The exercise is a continuous combination of movements of different positions to be completed without interruption. It is characterized not only by free, easy, flowing, bold and powerful rhythms, but also by mild, perfect, twining and continuous rhyme and meter. The movements are executed with a combination of hardness and softness, sometimes quickly and sometimes slowly, as the Yin and Yang supplement each other.

The starting position:

Stand with feet apart, slightly wider than shoulder width, tiptoe forward, and parallel to each other.

Points for attention: Keep the neck erect and head up, look straight ahead, with the chin tucked in. The face should look relaxed and natural. Relax the shoulders and keep the chest in, hands down by the sides, fingers slightly apart, palms empty, buttocks and anus contracted, legs slightly bent with the knees looking as if holding something between them. Keep the balls of the feet and toes on the ground, and use the mind to guide them into the ground like a big tree planting roots.

Then check the different parts of the body in the order described above for attention to be sure they are placed properly. Check them three times to discharge stale air from the body and let the fresh air flow in. By the way, if the starting exercise is done separately, it constitutes a still standing exercise, which is also beneficial to health.

The six-movement exercise:

[1] Strike the ears with both fists: Raise the arms from the sides of the body upward in curved lines to both sides, palms gradually turned down. At the same time, imagine sinking from the waist and hips, through the knees to the balls of the feet. Breathe in slowly and evenly. When the palms rise to shoulder level, turn the forearms inward, bend the arms slightly forward with the palms turned outward in a holding position, thumbs down, the other fingers forward, and the backs of the hands opposite each other like the wind striking the ears.

Continue the movement, continue to breathe in slowly and evenly, the radials between the thumbs and forefingers opposite each other at eye level, arms forming a big circle. (Fig. 8-39)

[2] The tiger crouches on the summit: Continue from the above movements, begin to breathe out evenly and slowly. Bend the arms back, withdraw the palms to the sides of the ears and change them into tiger's claws, fingers bending as if holding a round ball, shoulders dropped, elbows down, chest open and back straight. The *qi* (vital energy) now flows back to Dantian. (Fig. 8-40)

[3] Fierce tiger extends its claws: Continue from the above movements. Begin to breathe in evenly and slowly. Extend the tiger's claws forward, thumbs down, palms forward, forearms twisted inward, elbow joints down, chest in, back straight, wrist bent upward, elbows dropped, abdomen in, back straight, buttocks in and crotch tight. Look at the palms. (Fig. 8-41)

[4] Hungry tiger springs for food: Continue from the above movements, breathe in deeply, move the tiger's claws first downward and then inward (palms facing the lower abdomen), and then upward, roll the palms up in a curved line, bend the arms in a circle, hold the breath to conserve energy, and breathe out a bit. (Fig. 8-42)

[5] Push Mount Tai with all your might: Continue from the above movements. Turn the forearms inward powerfully, palms turned forward, shoulders dropped and elbows down, keep the palms up and push them forward at shoulder level, with *qi* (vital energy) flowing to the palm bases and the fingertips. At the same time, bend the knees quickly to crouch into a horse-riding stance, breathe out with the sound of "hey," waist sitting back, buttocks in and anus contracted. (Fig. 8-43)

Note: This movement should be executed with the mind, and not with force, but softly, slowly and relaxed if just for health pres-

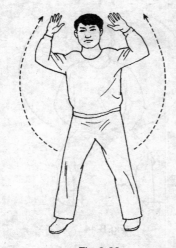

Fig. 8-39

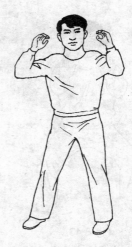

Fig. 8-40

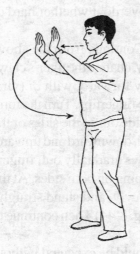

Fig. 8-41

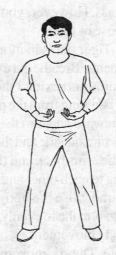

Fig. 8-42

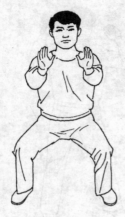

Fig. 8-43

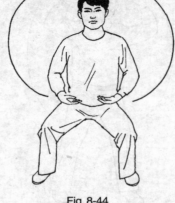

Fig. 8-44

ervation or medical treatment. If it is practised as a fighting skill, it should be executed quickly with toughness, power, fierceness and heaviness. However, you should never overdo it whether hard or soft, loose or tight.

[6] Tiger plays in mountain woods: Continue from the above movements. Breathe out evenly and slowly, change the tiger's claws into palms and extend them horizontally forward, with *qi* (vital energy) flowing from the palm bases to the fingertips. Turn the forearms outward and turn the palms from inside out so the sides of the thumbs turn outside and the palms forward, downward and upward. Bend the arms back and drop them, elbows gradually out, fingers pointing to each other and gradually dropping on both sides. At the same time, raise the body evenly and slowly, and stand straight. Begin to breathe in evenly and slowly.'(Fig. 8-44) Then continue to do the [1] movement.

Note: The six-movement exercise should be executed without interruption, with two inhalations and two exhalations. In doing the exercise, repeat it 9-36 times. The body rises and falls with continuous, uninterrupted movements. The breathing is even, slow and natural, and the movements are circular, lively and full.

Closing form: Continue to do the first through the sixth exercises. After changing to the form as shown in Fig. 8-39, turn the palms from forward to downward, and then drop the arms down evenly and slowly, breathe out evenly and slowly until both hands fall to the lower abdomen, with the internal energy flowing downward from the Baihui acupoint at top of the head to the Dantian acupoint at the abdomen. Continue to move the hands downward on both sides, and then back to the starting form. Finish the exercise after breathing 9 times at Dantian.

9. Patting exercise

The exercise of patting the whole body is a set of simple and easy movements. They help strengthen the tendons and bones, develop the muscles, improve the flexibility of the joints, promote the circulation of blood, and strengthen the functions and metabolism of the internal organs. In these exercises, you use your palms or fists to pat your whole body. After patting, you feel completely relaxed and cheerful, your movements become nimble and quick and your head refreshed. These exercises are more flexible and mobile than massage done by others, and therefore are more economical and effective.

The hands are generally used for these exercises, but some people use a steel swatter or sand bags to pat the body.

The exercise consist of eight parts:

[1] Pat the head

Description: In either standing form or walking form. When standing, relax the body, drop the shoulders and elbows, and pat the head with a smiling face. If walking, walk slowly and pat the head while walking, without any restraint.

Use the left palm to pat the left side of the head and the right palm to pat the right side of the head. Pat the head 50 times on each side. (Fig. 8-45) Then use the left palm to pat the other side of the inclined head and the right palm to do the same, 50 times each. Count the number of times in your mind, keep calm and breathe naturally. (Fig. 8-46)

Effect: Perseverance in doing the exercise helps prevent and cure dizziness, headache and the insufficient supply of blood to the brain.

[2] Pat the arms

Description: The same starting form as above. Use the right palm or fist to pat four sides of the left arm from above downward, 25 times on each side (in five groups, five times in each group). Then use the left palm or fist to pat the right arm in the same way. Pat 100-200 times in all, on the four sides. (Figs. 8-47, 8-48)

Effect: This helps relieve numbness and partial paralysis of the arms.

[3] Pat the shoulders

Description: The same starting form as above. First use the right palm to pat the left shoulder and then the left palm to pat the right shoulder. Pat the shoulders alternately 50 to 100 times each. (Figs. 8-49, 8-50)

Effect: This helps prevent and cure peripheral inflammation of the shoulder joints, cold shoulder, and poor muscle development.

[4] Pat the back

Description: The same starting form as above. First use the right fist to pat the left side of the back and then the left fist to pat the right side of the back, 100-200 times each. (Figs. 8-51, 8-52)

[5] Pat the chest

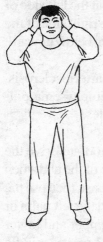

Fig. 8-45

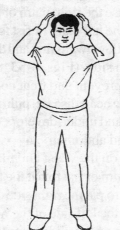

Fig. 8-46

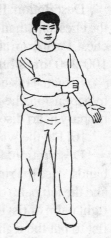

Fig. 8-47

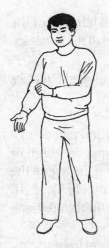

Fig. 8-48

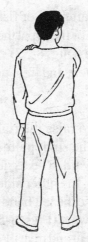

Fig. 8-49

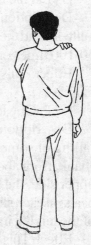

Fig. 8-50

Description: First use the right palm or fist to pat the left side of the chest and then use the left palm or fist to pat the right side of the chest. Pat it from above downward first and then from below upward, 100-200 times on each side. (Figs. 8-53, 8-54)

Effect: This helps prevent and treat coronary arteriosclerosis, hypertension, rheumatic heart disease, pulmonary emphysema, pulmonary heart disease, and under-developed muscles.

[6] Pat the waist and abdomen

Description: Pivot on the waist and turn the body to drive the hands. Use the right palm or fist to pat the left side of the abdomen and the left palm or fist to pat the right side of the waist, then use the right palm or fist to pat the left side of the waist and the left palm or fist to pat the right side of the abdomen. Pat the upper and lower parts of the abdomen with both hands, and pat the upper, middle and lower parts of the waist with both hands. Pat 100-200 times on each side. (Figs. 8-55, 8-56)

[7] Pat the buttocks

Description: Use the left palm or fist to pat the left side of the buttocks and the right palm or fist to pat the right side of the buttocks, 50-100 times on each side. (Fig. 8-57)

Effect: This helps prevent and treat poorly developed buttocks muscles.

[8] Pat the legs

Description: Stand and raise the right leg, with the heel on a railing of some sort, use the right palm or fist to pat the thigh or shank, from above downward, 5 beats at a time. Pat the leg on the upper side, the lower side, the outer side and the inner side, 5-10 beats on each side. Then use the left hand to pat the thigh and shank of the left leg in the same way. (Figs. 8-58, 8-59)

Effect: This helps prevent and treat ill-development leg muscles, partial paralysis, paraplegia, insensitivity in the legs, and general leg

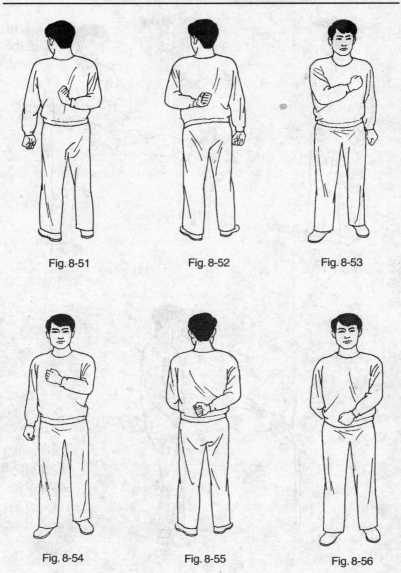

Fig. 8-51

Fig. 8-52

Fig. 8-53

Fig. 8-54

Fig. 8-55

Fig. 8-56

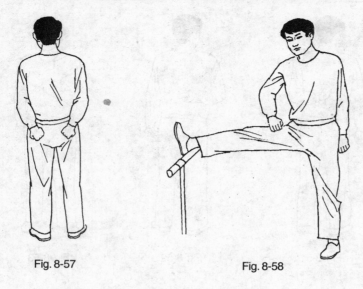

Fig. 8-57   Fig. 8-58

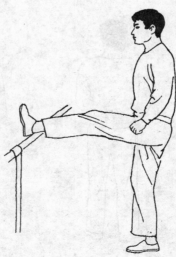

Fig. 8-59

weakness.

Points for attention: In patting the body, pat lightly at first and then heavily, and persevere.

10. Massaging exercises for preventing colds

The massaging exercises for preventing colds were worked out on the basis of the traditional Chinese medical use of acupuncture to treat colds.

According to the traditional Chinese medical theory of the meridian system, acupuncture at the Hegu, Yingxiang, Fengchi, Dazhui and Erchui acupoints helps prevent and treat colds, fever and cough. These exercises use the fingers and massage instead of needles to prevent and treat colds. Practice has shown that as long as you persevere, you will get satisfactory results.

The exercises consist of five parts:

[1] Rub the nose

Starting form: Cross the fingers and rub the thenars until they become warm.

Description: Use the right thenar to rub the right side of the nose, beginning from the base downward to Yingxiang and then use the left thenar to rub the left side of the nose in the same way. Rub both sides of the nose by using the hands alternately, 16 times each. (Fig. 8-60)

[2] Press the Hegu acupoints

Description: First use the right thumb to press Hegu on the left hand and turn-press it 16 times, and then use the left thumb to press Hegu on the right hand 16 times in the same way. (Fig. 8-61)

[3] Wash the face and pull the ears

Starting form: Rub the palms against each other until they are warm enough.

Description: Press the palms on the forehead and use both palms to rub down along the nose to the lower chin and then along the outer sides of the face upward. Use the thumbs and forefingers to pull the ears lightly to the outer sides when passing the ears, and then use the palms again to rub the face past the temples back to the forehead. Do this exercise 16 times. (Fig. 8-62)

[4] Massage the Yingxiang acupoints

Description: Use the cushions of both forefingers to rub the Yingxiang acupoints on both sides of the nose, 16 times on each side. (Fig. 8-63)

[5] Rub the Fengchi and Dazhui acupoints

Description: Use the three middle fingers of the right hand to rub the nape from the right Fengchi acupoint to the left Fengchi acupoint downward past the Dazhui acupoint and back to the right Fengchi. Repeat the exercise 8 times. Then use the left hand to do the exercise in the same way and repeat it 8 times. (Fig. 8-64)

The massaging exercises for the prevention of colds should be done once everyday. You will benefit as long as you do them with perseverance. You can increase the number of times for the whole set of exercise or a single exercise if you have cold symptoms. The preventive and curative effect will be even better if you do other physical exercises along with the massage.

11. "Rock-the-Sea" exercise

Rocking the sea is a self-massage exercise. If you learn it in the right way, it has a special curative effect for many diseases, including insomnia and stomach and intestinal disorders.

This is an exercise in which you sit quietly and turn and shake the upper part of your body gently and softly so that everything, including your internal organs, are exercised. This helps promote

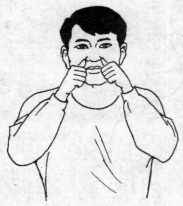

Fig. 8-60

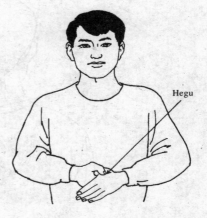

Hegu

Fig. 8-61

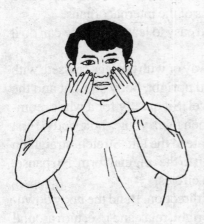

Fig. 8-62

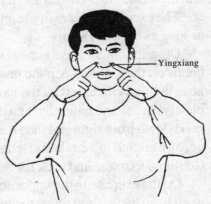

Yingxiang

Fig. 8-63

143

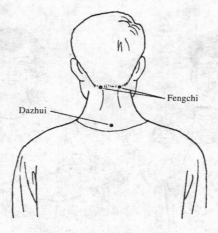

Fengchi

Dazhui

Fig. 8-64

the functions of the meridian system, regulate the circulation of blood and *qi*, and strengthen the functions of the internal organs.

The exercise is very simple and easy to learn. Anyone can do it as long as they can sit up.

Description: Sit in the normal way or with the legs crossed, with hands on the knees. Keep the head upright, body straight and the nose in line vertically with the navel. Sit quietly for a while, completely at ease and naturally, and then relax your whole body. First bend down from right and then rotate to the left. Stretch, straighten up, turn around in a circle and return to the original form. No pause. Continue to rotate and rock for 36 circles.

Do the exercise in the opposite direction. Bend the body downward from the left and rotate to the right, relax and rise, turn around in a circle and return to the original form. Rock in the same way for 36 circles. Return to the sitting position.

It is simple, but has a very good curative effect.

Points for attention:

[1] If the normal sitting position is used, it is best to sit on a wooden stool, feet apart to shoulder width and parallel to each other. An important point is to keep the outer sides of the feet parallel to each other.

[2] If you sit with legs crossed with the left leg above, you should rotate from right to left, and if the right leg is above, rotate from left to right.

[3] When you rotate with the upper body bent forward, pivot from the waist, with the nose in line vertically with the navel (be sure not to bend your head backward).

[4] The bending degree of the body while rotating depends on the illness and other individual circumstances. If you feel dizzy or depression in the chest, or have high blood pressure, the bending degree should not be too great; if you have a sore back, waist or limbs, the bending should be lower, and the bending should be moderate for gastric and intestinal disorders.

[5] Do these exercises slowly, evenly, relaxed and quietly, with the mind on the boundless sea and far-reaching sky as if you were rocking on the sea.

For medical treatment, do this several times a day and increase the number of times appropriately. If mainly for health preservation, you just rock your body 36 times from each side before going to bed, it takes about 15 minutes.

12. Iron crotch exercises

The iron crotch exercises are for improving physical fitness and treating illness.

This is a folk therapy for preventing and treating illness mainly by stimulating the scrotum. The testes in the scrotum secrete testosterone, the male hormone. Testosterone helps stimulate the normal development of the male sexual organs (including the epididymis, spermatic duct, ejaculatory duct, seminal vesicle, prostate and penis) and maintain their maturity. At the same time, it plays a decisive role in the emergence and maintenance of the male sexual character. It also has an important metabolic effect in stimulating muscle development.

So this hormone is extremely important. It is often used to treat illnesses, but if exercises are done as well, the physiological functions of the testis can be improved and the natural production of testosterone can be enhanced.

By persevering all year round, you can improve the functions of the testis, strengthen the penis and other sexual organs, and cure impotence and premature ejaculation.

There are many kinds of iron crotch exercises, but we will just recommend two sets that are simple and easy to learn:

The first set:

[1] Rub your hands warm, scoop your testis up with one hand and put the outer side of the little finger of the other hand by the fringe of the hair on the lower abdomen. Use both hands to scoop up and rub the testis and penis upward forcefully around 100 times. Then change hands to rub the testis and penis around 100 times.

A beginner should do the exercise lightly. After you have practised it for some time, you may exert more force and increase the number of times to hundreds. It depends on the individuals.

[2] Rub the hands warm first, and then rub the testis and penis back and forth with the proper force around 100 times.

[3] Use both palms to pinch the testis and penis and pull them up and down with force, 3-5 times.

[4] Use the fingers to rub the testis. Use the hands alternately, and rub the lower abdomen several dozen times.

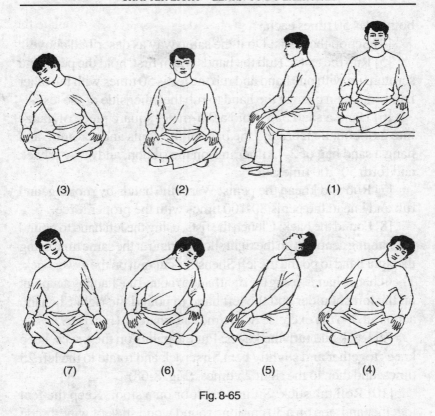

(3)　　　　　　　(2)　　　　　　　(1)

(7)　　　　(6)　　　　(5)　　　　(4)

Fig. 8-65

The second set:

[1] Push the abdomen downward: Place one hand on top of the other to push the abdomen from Jiantu point to the joint of the pubis, repeat 36 times. (Fig. 8-66)

[2] Rub the abdomen: Place one palm on top of the other and put them on the Qihai acupoint, first rub the abdomen counterclockwise 50 times, and then clockwise 50 times.

[3] Twist the spermatic ducts: Use the thumb, forefinger and middle finger to twist spermatic ducts at the base of the penis on

both sides 50 times each.

[4] Scoop the testis: Do it the same way as described above.

[5] Rub the testis: Rub the hands warm first, hold the penis and scrotum up with one hand and rub the testis 50 times with the other hand, and then change the hand to rub the other side of the testis.

[6] Hang a sand bag: Fold a 0.5-meter square piece of gauze into a ribbon, tie it around the base of the penis and scrotum, and hang a sand bag of 2-4 kilograms on the ribbon, and sway it back and forth 50-100 times.

[7] Rub and knead the penis: Warm the hands by rubbing, and rub and knead the penis 80-100 times with the proper force.

[8] Pound the back: Clench the fists, using the left hand to pound the Jianjing acupoint on the right shoulder and at the same time using the right hand to pound the left Shenshu acupoint on the lower back. Then change hands, using the right hand to pound the Jianjing acupoint on the left shoulder and the left hand to pound the right Shenshu acupoint. Do the exercise 8-16 times alternately. (Fig. 8-67)

[9] Rock and turn the knees: Put the palms on the knees, keep knees together and slightly bent, first rock and rotate to the left 25 times, and then to the right 25 times. (Fig. 8-68)

[10] Roll the stick: Sit in a chair or on a stool. Keep the feet together and step on a 30 cm-long round wood stick of wine-bottle size. Roll it 50 times. (Fig. 8-69)

[11] Pound the kidneys: Clench the fists, pound lightly on the Pishu, Shenshu and Zhishi acupoints 30-60 times respectively. Then warm them by rubbing, pressing and kneading.

Indications for the iron crotch exercises:

These exercises are most useful for older people and those who are physically weak. Once you learn them, it will help improve your health, make you strong, dispel illness and prolong life. It also has a very good curative effect for impotence, emission, premature

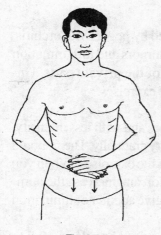

Fig. 8-66

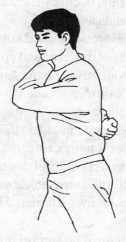

Fig. 8-67

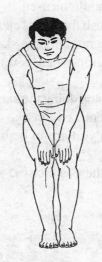

Fig. 8-68

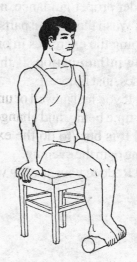

Fig. 8-69

ejaculation and decline of sexual function.

Contraindications:

These exercises should not be practised by pegde with orchitis, tuberculosis of the testis and epididymis, tumors and inflammation of the reproductive organs, and eczema of the private parts. Unmarried young men should not learn these exercises.

Points for attention:

[1] Beginners should do this fewer times and with less intensity, and increase the number of times and intensity gradually. There should be no pain or indication of discomfort after the exercises. When you become skillful, you should exert more effort and increase the number of times to several hundred in order to give adequate stimulation to the testis.

[2] You must be careful in hanging the sand bag. If you fail to grasp the essential points, something undesirable might happen. If not under proper guidance, no sand bags should be used.

[3] Wash the private parts frequently, wash the hands clean before doing the exercises in order to avoid scratching the skin and causing inflammation. If there is an erection when you do the exercises, just ignore it.

[4] If you feel unwell or uncomfortable, stop doing the exercises for the time being, and change to soft and gentle exercises.

[5] It is best to do the exercises when you are in bed in the morning or in the evening.

[6] Reduce your sex life when learning these exercises.

Chapter Nine
Self-Massage

Massage has a history of more than 2,000 years and is a treasured legacy of traditional Chinese medicine. Developed by the Chinese people over long years from ancient times, it has become an important component of traditional Chinese medicine.

China was one of the first countries to apply massage to medical care and treatment. Massage was already widely practised among the Chinese people as early as the Spring and Autumn and the Warring States periods, more than 2,000 years ago.

Massage is a passive physical exercise for health preservation. Traditional Chinese medicine believes that massage helps improve the meridian system, invigorate the circulation of blood and *qi* (vital energy) and activate the joints so as to regulate the balance between Yin and Yang and improve the functions of the internal organs. Modern medical research has also shown that massage helps regulate the function of the nervous system, improve the blood circulation and increase the body's resistance to disease.

Chinese massage has its own peculiarities, and is different from Western massage in content, technique and requirements. Traditional Chinese folk massage has the following characteristics:

[1] Chinese massage concentrates mainly on the acupoints, such as rubbing the Yongquan, pressing Yingxiang, kneading Dantian, and rubbing Fengchi acupoints. This was worked out on the basis of the theory of the meridian system in the light of symptoms by

distinguishing Yin from Yang and the empty from the solid. Western massage concentrates mainly on the muscles.

[2] It is guided by the medical theories of traditional Chinese medicine, and the theory of mutual help and the interrelationship between the heart and the kidneys, and stress is laid on the head and waist. Western massage stresses the four limbs.

[3] It employs the techniques of pounding and patting in most cases. For example, pounding the arms, patting the legs, beating the abdomen and waist, and there are more than a dozen techniques. Different techniques are used for different illnesses. Western massage mainly employs kneading and pinching.

[4] It calls for concentration, calm and a relaxed body while Western massage does not.

Self-massage is an exercise which combines both dynamic and still movements and is used for both preventive and curative purposes. It helps stimulate the acupoints and improve physical fitness, is simple and easy to do, and produces very good results.

The common techniques include:

Pressing: Use fingers, palm and the base of the hand to press a certain part with rising and falling motions. The pressing should be light at the beginning and become heavier, rhythmical, and elastic. The force should be reduced gradually at the end instead of stopping suddenly. The force is applied not only to the skin, but also to the muscle, bone and internal organs. The exercise helps to remove obstructions in the meridians, remove blood stasis and alleviate pain, and is applicable to all parts of the body.

Massaging: Put the cushions of the index finger, middle finger and ring finger, or the palm, on the skin to massage any part in a circular way with rhythms. Apply force mildly and naturally only to the skin and subcutaneous tissue. Generally, this method is used for the chest, abdomen, flanks and ribs. It helps regulate the peristalsis of the stomach and intestines, relax muscle tension, relieve swelling, remove blood stasis, regulate the flow of vital energy, invigorate the stomach, and remove food stagnation.

Pushing: Push forward and backward, or to the left and right on the skin in a straight line with the cushions of the fingers, palm, or base of the hand. While pushing, keep them close to the skin, apply force steadily and slowly. When less force is applied, it reaches only the subcutaneous tissue, but when greater force is applied, it reaches the muscles, and even the internal organs. The pushing exercise helps relax the muscles and tendons, and stimulate blood circulation, relieve inflammation, alleviate pain, and dispel fatigue.

Kneading: Knead certain acupoints lightly, softly and mildly in a circular way with the cushions of the fingers or the palm. Keep the hands close to the skin. The range of kneading depends on size and body weight and the tightness of the skin. It helps to remove obstructions in the channels and collaterals of the meridian system, stimulate blood circulation to remove blood stasis, relieve swelling and alleviate pain.

Foulaging: Rub and twist the skin back and forth quickly and forcefully with both palms or the fingers of both hands to warm the skin and subcutaneous tissue. This helps dispel wind and cold, promote blood flow to remove blood stasis, relax the muscles, and invigorate the kidneys.

Rubbing: Rub certain parts back and forth in a straight line with the palms or thenars at an even speed. Keep the hands close to the skin instead of applying pressure. This method is usually used for the chest, abdomen, waist and limbs. It helps remove obstructions in the channels and collaterals of the meridian system, relieve swelling, alleviate pain, and invigorate the spleen and stomach.

Grasping: Grasp and knead the skin, muscles or tendons of certain parts with the thumb, index finger and middle finger or with four fingers, with force applied first lightly and then heavily, but evenly and continuously. This helps remove obstructions in the channels and collaterals of the meridian system, alleviate muscle fatigue, and strengthen the muscles.

Points for attention:

[1] Choose an appropriate time to do the exercises, usually in the morning or before going to bed. It is best to do self-massage in a room with a moderate temperature and fresh air.

[2] Concentrate the mind and keep the surroundings quiet. And keep your hands clean and warm.

[3] Self-massage should be done directly on the skin. Ask a family member to help massage parts which you cannot reach yourself.

[4] The handwork should be light and soft, first light and later heavy, first shallow and later deep, with moderate force applied.

[5] Do not massage the abdomen, waist and sacrum, or the Hegu, Sanyinjiao, Kunlun and Jianjing acupoints of a pregnant woman.

[6] Stop self-massage on any parts of the body with acute inflammation, eczema, ulcers, boils, tumors or injuries.

1. Forty self-massage exercises for health protection

Doing self-massage exercises earnestly in the following order in the morning or before going to bed in the evening every day not only helps improve physical fitness and prolong life, but also may cure some chronic diseases. However, only perseverance produces good results (it takes 30 minutes to do all 40 exercises). Refer to Fig. 9-1 and Fig. 9-2 for the acupoints.

Breathe deeply 10 times before self-massaging to get rid of the stale and take in the fresh, and promote the circulation of vital en-

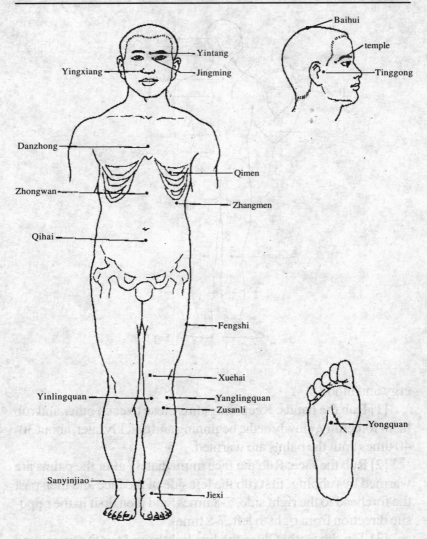

Fig. 9-1

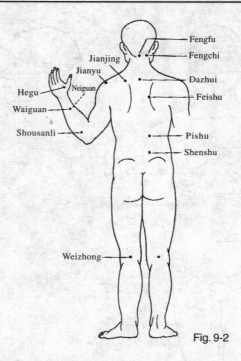

Fig. 9-2

ergy and blood.

[1] Rub the hands: Keep the palms close to each other and rub them forcefully, slowly at the beginning and quickly later, about 30-40 times until the palms are warmed.

[2] Rub the face: Rub the face immediately after the palms are warmed by rubbing, first rub the left side of the face and then past the forehead to the right side, 7-8 times, and then do it in the opposite direction from right to left, 7-8 times.

[3] Tap the teeth: Close the lips lightly and tap the upper and lower teeth together with rhythm, 30-40 times.

[4] Stir the tongue: Move the tongue up and down and right to

left between the teeth and lips, and left to right, 30 times each.

[5] Vibrate the ears: Keep the four fingers at the back of the head and the palms on the ears, and then vibrate the ears quickly and rhythmically about 30-40 times.

[6] Sound the celestial drum: Cover the ears with the base of the palms to keep air from the ears with the fingers on the back of the head. Press the cushions of the fore fingers on the back of the middle fingers and slip forefingers down to knock the back of the head with the sound of rub-a-dab. Snap the fingers 10-20 times.

[7] Rub Jingming: First rub the Yintang acupoint 20 times with fingers, then massage the eye sockets 10 times each with both hands, and finally rub both Jingming acupoints 20 times at the same time.

[8] Rub the temples: Rub and press the temples with both hands 20 times.

[9] Wipe the forehead: Wipe the forehead with both hands 20 times.

[10] Push Yingxiang: Push the Yingxiang acupoints on both sides of the nose with hands 20 times.

[11] Push Tinggong: Push the Tinggong acupoints 20 times with both hands.

[12] Massage the cheeks: Rub the cheeks with both hands 20 times.

[13] Knead Baihui: Knead the Baihui acupoint with both hands, 20 times each.

[14] Press Fengchi: Press and knead the Fengchi acupoints on the two sides with the hands 20 times each.

[15] Press Dazhui: Press the Dazhui acupoint 20 times with each hand.

[16] Knead Feishu: Press and knead the Feishu acupoints on both sides with each hand 20 times.

[17] Knead Pishu: Press and knead the Pishu acupoints on both

157

sides with each hand 20 times.

[18] Knead Shenshu: Rub and knead the Shenshu acupoints on both sides with each hand 40 times.

[19] Knead the Danzhong: Knead the Danzhong acupoint with each hand 20 times.

[20] Knead Zhongwan: Knead the Zhongwan acupoint with each hand 20 times.

[21] Knead the Qihai: Knead the Qihai acupoint with each hand 30 times.

[22] Rub the upper chest: Rub the upper part of the chest 20 times with each hand.

[23] Pat the chest: Keep the fingers apart and pat the chest 7-10 times with the front of the fingers. Breathe in while patting.

[24] Rub Zhangmen: Rub the Zhangmen acupoints with both hands 30 times at the same time.

[25] Rub the lower abdomen: Rub the lower part of the abdomen with both hands, 30 times each.

[26] Knead Jianjing: Grasp and knead the left Jianjing acupoint with right hand, and the right Jianjing with left hand 20 times each.

[27] Knead Jianyu: Grasp and knead the left Jianyu point with the right hand, and the right Jianyu with the left hand, 20 times each.

[28] Grasp Shousanli: Grasp and knead the Shousanli acupoints with the opposite hand, 20 times each.

[29] Grasp Neiguan and Waiguan: Grasp and knead the Neiguan and Waiguan acupoints of one hand with the other hand, 10 times each acupoint.

[30] Knead Hegu: Grasp and knead the Hegu acupoints with the opposite hand 20 times each.

[31] Foulage the arms: Foulage the arms with the opposite hand, 10 times each.

[32] Twist the fingers: Twist and rub all fingers three times.

[33] Press Fengshi: Point-press the Fengshi acupoints with both hands, 20 times each.

[34] Knead Xuehai: Knead and press the Xuehai acupoints with both hands, 10 times each.

[35] Grasp Lingquan: Grasp the Yin and Yang Lingquan acupoints on both sides of each leg with both hands, 10 times each acupoint.

[36] Press Zusanli: Press and knead the Zusanli acupoints with both hands, 20 times each.

[37] Knead Sanyinjiao: Press and knead the Sanyinjiao acupoints with both hands, 20 times each.

[38] Beat the legs: Clench the fists to beat the legs, 10 times each.

[39] Foulage the legs: Foulage and knead the legs with both hands, 20 times respectively.

[40] Rub Yongquan: Knead and rub the Yongquan acupoints on the soles of both feet with the fingers, 20 times respectively.

2. Head massage for hypertension sufferers

Hypertension occurs mostly among middle-aged and older people. Common symptoms are headache and dizziness. Besides medication, self-massage on the head also helps treat hypertension as it dilates the blood vessels and promotes the circulation of blood and aids metabolism.

Self-massage on the head consists of the following 13 exercises:

[1] Comb the hair: First stroke the head with both palms five times and then bend the fingers to comb the hair with the fingernails. Separate the hair from the middle of the top, comb the left half of the head with the left hand and the right half of the head with the right hand. Comb five times on each side as a unit, and comb 10 units in all.

[2] Wash the face: Rub the palms warm first and then wash the face from the top of the forehead down to the lower jaw with both hands. Wash the left side of the face with the left hand and the right side of the face with the right hand. Moving the hand up and down counts as once, and wash the face 10 times in all.

[3] Massage the top of the head: Put both palms on the top of the head, with the middle fingers at the Baihui acupoint. Start at Baihui, massage from the top of the head to the Yintang acupoint with both hands, separate the hands, the middle finger of the left hand along the left eyebrow to the corner of the eye, and the middle finger of the right hand along the right eyebrow to the corner of the eye. Do this 10 times.

[4] Twist and point-press the temples: Point-press and twist the temples with the thumbs of both hands. Point-press at the temples with the fingertips and twist in a circle. One circle counts as once. Do this 10 times.

[5] Point-press the Fengchi: Put the thumbs on the temples, with the other fingers on the head, move the thumbs from the temples along the ear roots to the Fengchi acupoints behind the ears. Point-press and twist Fenchi with both thumbs. Do it 10 times.

[6] Point-press Fengfu: Put the right thumb at the Fengfu acupoint, the other fingers on the head, so as to fix the head. Then point-press Fengfu with the right thumb and at the same time use the thumb to draw a circle. One circle counts as once. Do it this way 10 times. Then change to the left thumb to point-press Fengfu in the same way 10 times.

[7] Pat and knead the large muscles of the neck: First grasp the muscle of the neck with the left palm, grasp and knead it with force, kneading and letting go alternately. Do it 10 times. Then change to the right palm, and do the same 10 times.

[8] Massage the helix: Put the thumbs at the back of the ears,

and the index fingers in the auricles, press and knead the ears from both inside and outside in the opposite directions, from above downward to seek the aching points. After the aching points are found, press the fingers on the points and massage the points in the pressure-reducing grooves 10 times (Fig. 9-3)

[9] Rap the head: Bend the fingers of both hands into a right angle, start from the mid-point of the head and use the fingernails of the left hand to knock the left side of the head and the right fingernails to knock the right side of the head, from above to below, from left to right, and from front to back, and knock the head all over. This counts as once. Do this 10 times.

[10] Grasp and knead the shoulder muscles: Grasp and knead the muscle (the highest part of the shoulder) of the right shoulder with the left hand 10 times, change to the right hand to grasp the muscle of the left shoulder 10 times. Massage the left and right sides with the palms 10 times each after grasping and kneading.

[11] Relax the muscles of the armpits: Knead the muscle in the middle of the right armpit with the left hand 10 times and change to the right fingers to knead the muscle in the middle of the left armpit

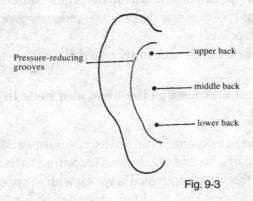

Pressure-reducing grooves

upper back

middle back

lower back

Fig. 9-3

10 times. Finally, massage both armpits with fingers 10 times each.

[12] Knead Weizhong: Grasp and knead the muscle at the Weizhong acupoint at the back of the right knee with left fingers 10 times, and use the right fingers to grasp and knead the muscle at the Weizhong acupoint at the back of the left knee 10 times. Finally, massage Weizhong with fingers 10 times each.

[13] Point-press Yongquan: Use the thumb to point-press the Yongquan acupoint in the depression of the sole. Knead and point-press Yongquan while drawing a circle with the thumb. Do this on each foot 10 times.

Points for attention:

Wash the head and face clean, dry them, have all fingernails cut smoothly and wash the hands clean before doing these exercises. Do not use strong force in point-pressing and massaging the acupoints. The handwork should be light at first and become heavy later. Do not damage the skin and soft tissues. If the parts to be massaged are afflicted, do not massage them to avoid damage and infection.

The indications for these exercises are hypertension, cerebral arteriosclerosis, hypertension, and neurosis. Those suffering from hyrotension should not massage the pressure-reducing grooves and the Yongquan acupoints.

Do this set of exercises once or twice a day.

3. Rub the soles and massage the head and neck to reduce blood pressure

Hypertension is a common cardiovascular ailment. Its main symptoms are headache and dizziness. According to traditional Chinese medical theory "if something is wrong with an upper part of the body, give treatment first to a lower part of the body," so self-massage should be used to reduce the blood pressure by rubbing and kneading the Yongquan acupoints on the soles. This method has the function of reducing everything. Traditional Chinese medicine calls massage at these two acupoints the method of "taking away the firewood from under the cauldron" or "conducting the fire back to its origin." Rubbing the soles helps reduce the liver heat, conduct the blood flow downward, and lighten the burden on the head, thus alleviating headache and dizziness. Moreover, traditional Chinese medicine also believes that massaging the head and neck, especially pushing and massaging the pressure-reducing grooves and the cervical artery behind the ears, helps direct the downward flow of the blood in the head and weaken the upsurging force of blood, thus refreshing the brain and improving eyesight.

Of course, there are many factors that cause hypertension and medical treatment should be applied in many ways. If self-massage is added to drug treatment, acupuncture and diet therapy, the effect will be much better. Self-massage for reducing blood pressure is very simple and easy to do. Hypertension sufferers should try it for some time.

This is how to do it:

[1] Rub the soles: Before getting up in the morning and going to bed in the evening drape a garment over your shoulders, sit on the bed, and rub the Yongquan acupoints on your soles with your thumbs (Fig. 9-1) 100 times each (about two minutes). Or rub and knead the right sole with the left heel and rub and knead the left sole with the right heel, 100 times each. Mind you, rub toward the toes forcefully, not back and forth.

[2] Massage the head and neck: Start with both palms pushing and massaging the head from the forehead backward to the occipital bone. Then, turn the palms up and use the outer sides of the small fingers to push and massage from above the ear downward to the

pressure-reducing grooves (Fig. 9-3) behind the ears to the Fengchi acupoints (Fig. 9-2). Finally, use the sides of the back of the hands to push and massage the cervical artery downward to the front of the chest. This exercise takes about half a minute.

These two exercises can be done continuously at the same time. Rub and massage the head and neck after rubbing the soles or rub the soles after massaging the head and neck. Usually, you fell relaxed in head and the blood pressure reduced by 10-20 mm after the exercises, and this will last 4 to 5 hours. To consolidate the curative effect, massage the head and neck any time you wish.

This method is easy to follow, but it calls for perseverance for satisfactory results. Moreover, you should take some oral medicines at the beginning. As time goes on, cut down the dosage gradually under the guidance of a doctor in light of the drop in blood pressure.

4. Point-pressing therapy, massage and functional exercises for cervical vertebra diseases.

Cervical vertebra disease is common among middle-aged and older people. Those whose cases are not serious suffer from pain and numbness in the head, neck, shoulders, arms or hands, while those whose cases are serious have muscle atrophy or may be paralyzed and unable to take care of themselves.

The external factors causing cervical vertebra diseases are attacks by wind, cold, dampness or pathogenic agents, causing the stagnation of *qi* (vital energy) and blood. The internal factors are the gradual decline of the liver and kidney and the accompanied degeneration of the muscles and bones.

Treatment of the cervical vertebra diseases in traditional Chinese medicine includes, apart from the application of oral and local medication, point-pressing therapy, self-massage and functional exercises used to broaden the space between the vertebrae, make the cervical vertebrae nimble, and alleviate nerve pressure, thus relieving muscle tension and spasms, improving blood circulation, and metabolism of the bones and the resilience of the ligaments of the muscles around the cervical vertebrae.

Middle-aged and older sufferers of cervical vertebra disease are advised to do the following for self-treatment. Those who do not suffer from this disease may as well have a try for preventive purposes.

Point-pressing therapy for sores, numbness and pain in the hands:

[1] Point-press the Hegu acupoint on the aching side with the thumb for 30 seconds. (Fig. 9-4)

[2] Point-press the Yangchi acupoint on the aching side with the thumb and middle finger for 30 seconds. (Fig. 9-5)

[3] Tap and poke the Quchi acupoint on the aching side with the thumb for 30 seconds. (Fig. 9-6)

[4] Tap and poke the Shaohai acupoint on the aching side with the index and middle fingers for 30 seconds. (Fig. 9-7)

[5] Point-press the Quepeng acupoint on the aching side slowly with the thumb and middle finger for 1 minute. (Fig. 9-8)

[6] Point-press the Jianjing acupoint on the aching side with the index, middle and ring fingers for 1 minute. (Fig. 9-9)

[7] Tap and poke the Fengchi acupoint on the aching side with the middle and index fingers for 1 minute. (Fig. 9- 10)

[8] Point-press the Wan'gu acupoint on the aching side with the middle finger for 1 minute. (Fig. 9-11)

Self-massage for the neck:

[1] First massage the muscles on the aching side of the neck lightly from above to below with the index, middle, ring and little fingers, then use both hands to massage the muscles on both sides of the neck for 1 or 2 minutes.

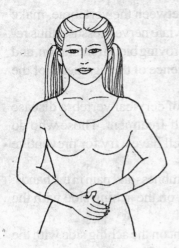

Fig. 9-4

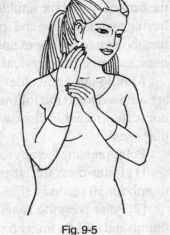

Fig. 9-5

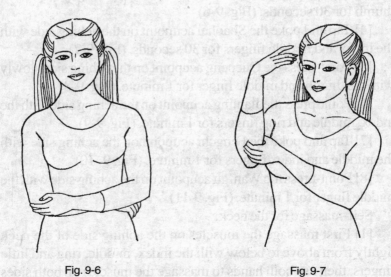

Fig. 9-6

Fig. 9-7

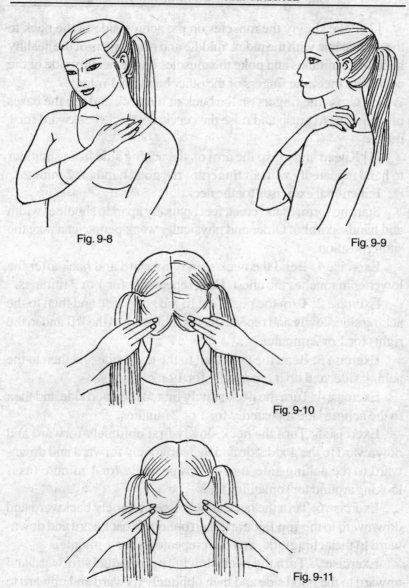

Fig. 9-8

Fig. 9-9

Fig. 9-10

Fig. 9-11

167

[2] Poke slowly the muscles on the aching side of the neck to the middle line with the index, middle and ring fingers of the healthy hand for 2 minutes and poke the muscles on the healthy side of the neck with the same fingers of the other hand for 1 minute.

[3] Cross the fingers on the back of the neck and use the bases of the palms to grasp and raise the cervical muscle backward for 1 minute.

[4] Knead and grasp the arm on the aching side from shoulder to hand repeatedly with all fingers of the good hand for 2 minutes.

Functional exercises for the neck:

Starting form: Stand erect, feet naturally apart to shoulder width and hands akimbo. Older and physically weak people can take the sitting position.

Exercise 1: Bend the neck slowly forward and back after the lower chin touches the chest. Do it repeatedly for 1 or 2 minutes.

Exercise 2: Turn the neck first to the good side and then to the aching side slowly and repeatedly (as if looking to the left and to the right) for 1 or 2 minutes.

Exercise 3: Bend the neck first to the good side and then to the aching side, and do it repeatedly for 1 or 2 minutes.

Exercise 4: Turn the neck slowly first to the good side and then to the aching side repeatedly for 1 or 2 minutes.

Exercise 5: Turn the neck slowly first obliquely forward and downward to the good side and then obliquely forward and downward to the aching side, and do it repeatedly for 1 minute (as if looking around for something).

Exercise 6: Turn the neck slowly first obliquely backward and downward to the good side and then obliquely backward and downward to the aching side, and do it repeatedly for 1 minute.

Exercise 7: Turn the neck slowly first obliquely forward and upward to the good side and then obliquely forward and upward to

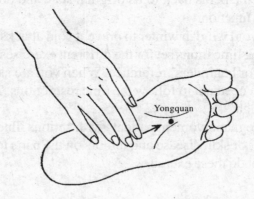

Fig. 9-33

shirt and underpants.

[2] When doing the exercises, close the eyes slightly, concentrate the mind, lick the upper palate with the tongue, and with palms against the skin. Connect one exercise with another and apply force moderately. It is desirable to have the whole body warm and sweating lightly when the whole set of exercises is finished.

[3] When massaging the Yingxiang, Fengchi and Jianjing acupoints, apply some force so that the massaged parts feel sore. When massaging the waist and back, you can take a break before finishing it if you do not have enough arm power.

[4] After finishing the last exercise, men should cup the scrotum with the hand, massage it by rotating downward, and reduce stimulation to the penis as much as possible. If some beginners have an erection and cannot return to the normal state in a short time after massage, they can use their middle fingers to point-press the Guanyuan acupoint in the midpoint on the lower abdomen, 10 cm under the navel, apply force inward slowly for 2 minutes. This

helps put the penis back to its original state and does no harm to the sexual function.

[5] Avoid wind in winter to prevent cold attacks.

[6] The time limits set for the different exercises in description are only for beginners' reference. When you are skilled in doing them, you need not to follow the time restrictions. Ten minutes is quite enough.

[7] Pregnant women, patients with serious illnesses or with a high fever or skin disease and tumors on the parts to be massaged should not do these exercises.

Chapter Ten

Ways to Improve Health Without Taking Drugs

The art of preserving health has a recorded history of more than 3,000 years in China. Since ancient times, China has had a set of methods for health improvement without drugs, including acupuncture, massage, qigong and Taiji Quan. As they are simple, practical and effective, and have no side effects, they are still very popular and widely practised even today when modern medicine is highly developed.

1. Finger-pressing therapy for treating common and frequently occurring diseases among older people

When people grow old, some common diseases frequently occur. It is very useful to learn this finger-pressing therapy which helps to solve certain problems. Older people might have a try.

[1] Headache: Headache is mostly caused by wind-cold, colds, sequelae of cerebral thrombus, spasms of cerebral blood vessels and neurosis.

When the finger-pressing therapy is applied, press the Lieque acupoints. The acupoints are located on the radial sides of both forearms, proximal to the styloid process of the radius, about three-finger width above the crease of the wrist. (Fig. 10-1)

Description: Point-pressing the acupoint with the thumb. If you have a headache on the left side, point-pressing Lieque on the right arm, and if you have a headache on the right side, point-pressing Lieque on the left arm. If you have a severe headache, point-pressing the acupoints on both arms. While doing it, keep on moving the pressing thumb until you feel sore and heavy. The time for point-pressing is about 1 minute, and stop pressing when the headache disappears. You can also point-pressing to the temples at the same time. (Fig. 10-2)

[2] Dizziness: Dizziness is common among older people. Heatstroke, carsickness and seasickness can also cause dizziness.

When applying the finger-pressing therapy, it should be applied to the Yintang point, located on the forehead at the midpoint in the line between the eyebrows near the nose. (Fig. 10-2)

Description: Point-pressing the acupoint with the index or middle finger, and move the finger horizontally. It is effective when the facial skin feels sore and numb. In order to make it more effective, point-pressing the Renzhong and Baihui acupoints at the same time.

[3] Toothache: Toothache often arises from the acute inflammation of the oral cavity due to excessive internal heat, dental caries, exposure of the tooth nerve and swollen of the gums.

Point-pressing the Hegu acupoint, located in the depressions between the first and second metacarpal bones on the back of both hands. (Fig. 10-3)

Description: Press the Hegu acupoint with the thumb, and move it up and down. Click the lower and upper teeth together at the same time. Stop pressing when the pain disappears. Press the acupoint on the right hand when the toothache is on the left side, and press the left hand when the toothache is on the right side. If you have toothache all over, apply point-pressure to both hands. Also, when you have an ache in an upper tooth, point-pressure way also be applied to the Jiache acupoints on the cheeks. (Fig. 10-4)

[4] Tinnitus: Tinnitus often causes people trouble. It can disturb

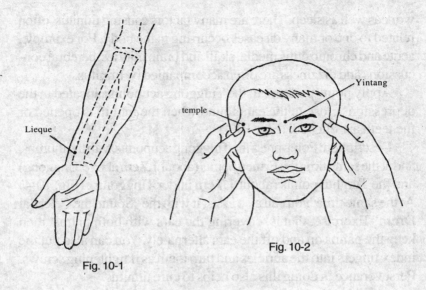

Lieque

Yintang

temple

Fig. 10-1

Fig. 10-2

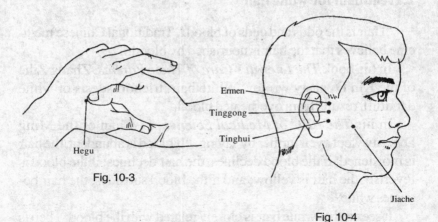

Ermen

Tinggong

Tinghui

Hegu

Fig. 10-3

Jiache

Fig. 10-4

work as well as sleep. There are many factors causing tinnitus, often related to one or many diseases occurring in the body. For example, acute and chronic otitis media, skull and brain injuries, cerebral concussions and dizziness are often accompanied by tinnitus.

Apply point-pressure to the Tinggong acupoints, located in the depressions close to the ears found when the mouth is opened or the teeth are clicked. (Fig. 10-4)

Description: Point-press the Tinggong acupoints with the thumbs, and at the same time the Ermen points (about 1.7 cm above Tinggong) and the Tinghui points (about 1.7 cm under Tinggong). (Fig. 10-4) At the same time, you can also assist it with the "Sound the Celestial Drum" Exercise, that is, covering the ears with both palms, then keep the palms on and off the ears alternately. You can also put the index fingers into the auricles and turn them as if tightening screws. Perseverance in doing this also helps to cure tinnitus.

2. Treatment for white hair

"Hair is the odds and ends of blood." Traditional Chinese medicine believes that the hair is nourished by blood.

In his book *The Literati's Care of Their Parents*, Zhang Zihe of the Kin Dynasty wrote: "White hair, trichomadesis or white dandruff results from overheated blood."

In his *The ABC of Medical Science*, Li Chan of the Ming Dynasty went even further by saying: "If blood is abundant, the hair is moistened; if the blood declines, the hair declines; if the blood is feverish, the hair is yellow; and if the blood subsides, the hair becomes white."

It seems that white hair is closely related with the blood. Then is there anything that can be done to blacken white hair? The answer is yes. According to the medical books, the physical and breathing exercises which ancient Chinese called "dao yin" can remove the obstruction in the circulation of *qi* (vital energy) and blood and is very beneficial for the treatment of this condition.

[1] The following is described in a book compiled by Zhou Lujing during the Ming Dynasty:

At 1:00 in early morning and 12:00 at noon, sit up straight, hand in hand, concentrate the mind, dispel all distracting thoughts, both eyes looking internally at the top of the head, and you naturally find both the Yin *qi* and Yang *qi* rise up from the sacrum along the spinal column to the top of the head. It then flows down to the nose, the lower chin and throat, and then along the midline of the chest and abdomen to the Dantian point 10 cm below the navel. Doing this nine times will make you vigorous and filled with *qi* and blood, and white hair will become black again.

[2] In another book *The General Treatise on the Etiology and Symptomology of the Diseases-Origin of White Hair* under the heading "Formula of Health Preservation, Dao Yin Exercises," three methods are described.

a. After getting up in the morning, raise the right hand and put it across the head to grasp the left ear, and then raise the left hand and put it across the head to grasp the right ear. Lift the ears up with the hands simultaneously. (Fig. 10-6) Then keep on lifting the hair and beard with the hands. This helps to stimulate the circulation of *qi* and blood in the beard and hair.

b. Sit on the ground, stretch the legs, stretch the hands, fingers toward the insteps, and double the body, head touching the ground. (Fig. 10-7) This method helps invigorate the spinal column, promote the circulation of *qi* and blood in the roots of the hair, and keep the hair good for a long time. Then, sit on a stool, relax the legs, keep the feet 30 cm apart, hold the smallest parts of the shanks just above the ankles with the hands, and double the body, head touching the ground. Do this 12 times. (Fig. 10-8) Invigorating the spinal column this way helps keep people well and directs the vital energy to moisten the hair so that it can grow well and remain black, soft and shining.

c. Bend the knees in a sitting position, the hips not touching the ground and the thighs and shanks forming right angles. Double the body, grasp the toes of both feet with the hands and keep them upward. Then lower the head and keep it as near to the ground as possible. (Fig. 10-9) This exercise helps transmit the vital energy from the heart, liver, spleen, lungs and kidneys fully to the head. It can cure deafness and dim sight. Perseverance in doing the exercise for a long time will turn white hair black again.

[3] The book *Da Tong Lei Ju Fang* says: "Black hair results from abundance of blood. Comb it once a day." *The Book of Prolonging Life* says: "The combing of the hair is often counted to 120." In other words, the hair should be combed very often. Of course, it is not limited to once a day and 120 strokes at a time. Frequent combing is beneficial to the scalp and hair roots, and helps promote the metabolism. (Fig. 10-10)

In fact, scalp massage is even more effective than combing the hair. Before going to bed or after getting up in the morning, massage the head by drawing small circles on the scalp with the index and middle fingers, from the forehead past the top of the head to the back of the head, and then from the forehead past the temples on the two sides to the back of the head. Massage it twice a day, 10-15 minutes a time. Rub and knead the scalp 30-40 times per minute. Perseverance in doing this year round will produce good effects. (Fig. 10-11)

Because massaging the scalp helps promote blood circulation, it enables the hair papilla to get more nutriments and increase the production of melanin, and at the same time remove obstructions from

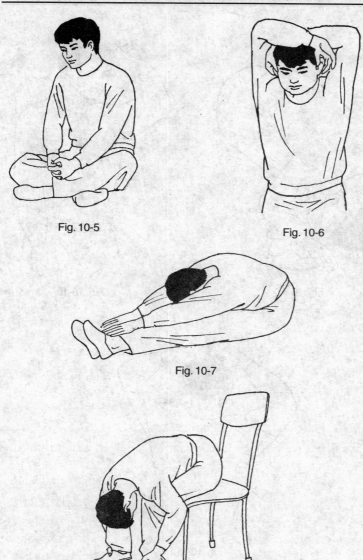

Fig. 10-5

Fig. 10-6

Fig. 10-7

Fig. 10-8

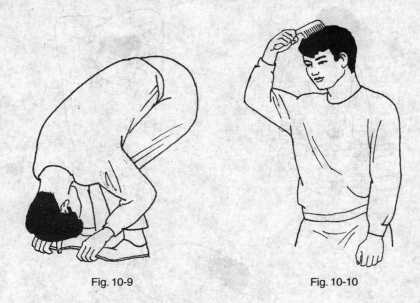

Fig. 10-9

Fig. 10-10

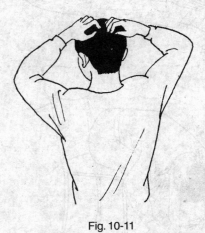

Fig. 10-11

the channels for the transmission of melanin, thus turning white hair black again.

3. Cure for stiff neck

Many people experience stiff neck after sleep. When you have a stiff neck, you find it difficult to tolerate the pain in the neck and cannot turn your head. If you turn your trunk with a stiff neck, the pain is even more acute, and sometimes the pain even extends to the shoulders and back.

The main cause of stiff neck is over-fatigue. If the pillow is too high when you sleep, it overstretches some muscles (mainly the sternocleidomastoid and trapezius) for a long time, thus causing the stasis of vital energy and blood. In some cases, This is because one reads or works by bending the head for too long, causing strain to the muscle group at the back of the neck, or an abrupt twist of the head that may also cause strain to the neck muscle.

Generally, a stiff neck will recur if preventive measures are not taken. People suffering from cervical vertebra diseases often have stiff necks.

Stiff neck can be prevented. The traditional Chinese way to prevent it is to practise Taijiquan, and other exercises. The "Cloud Hand" movement in Taiji, is very helpful in preventing stiff neck.

However, stiff neck is not regarded by people as an illness. Usually, stiff neck sufferers would drag on for a few days before going to a doctor only when the pain becomes unbearable. This is not good. If you do the exercises in good time, it will help you recover quickly.

Physical exercise therapy is generally done in two steps:

First step: Do not be afraid of the pain, but draw the strained muscle in the neck slowly toward the obstructed direction. Turn the neck repeatedly. The sufferers should first point-pressing the affected point and massage it with the thumb, and then press and knead the painful muscle with the palm. At the same time, turn the head, bend it forward or backward toward the direction in which you turn with pain.

Second step: After the neck is somewhat improved, do the following exercises for the prevention and treatment of stiff neck and cervical vertebra diseases:

(1) Clench the fists and bend the elbows

Starting form: Stand naturally with arms down.

Movements: [1] Clench the fists and bend the elbows at the same time. Stretch the arms backward powerfully. (Fig. 10-12) [2] Return to the starting form.

(2) Bend forward and backward

Starting form: Stand naturally with hands akimbo.

Movements: [1] Bend the head forward and then bend the body backward slowly and as far as possible. (Fig. 10-13) [2] Return to the starting form.

(3) Thrust fists obliquely forward

Starting form: Clench the fists, elbows bent at a right angle, and stand with feet apart.

Movements: [1] Turn the body to the right and thrust the left fist to the right, and return to the starting form. [2] Turn to the left and thrust the right fist to the left, and return to the starting form. (Fig. 10-14)

(4) Turn the head to both sides

Starting form: Stand with feet apart, hands akimbo.

Movements: [1] Turn the head to the right, and return to the starting form. [2] Turn the head to the left, and return to the starting form. (Fig. 10-15)

(5) Hold up the sky with both hands

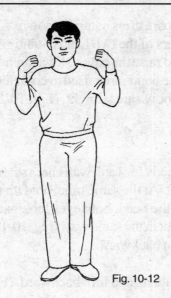

Fig. 10-12

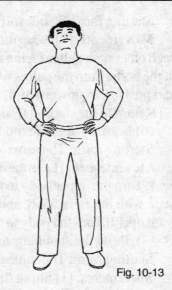

Fig. 10-13

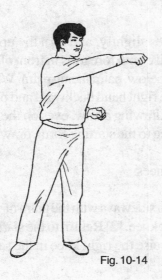

Fig. 10-14

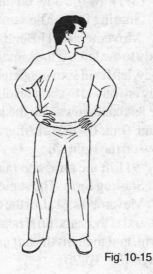

Fig. 10-15

Starting form: Stand with feet apart, arms naturally down.

Movements: [1] Keep the fingers of the two hands pointing to each other with palms facing up, and raise the hands slowly in front of the body. Turn the palms when the hands are raised to chest level and push them upward until the elbows are straight. (Fig. 10-16) [2] Return to the starting form.

(6) Look back at the moon

Starting form: The same as (5).

Movements: [1] Lean the upper body forward, with knees slightly bent. Turn the upper body to the left. At the same time, hold up the neck with the right hand, and turn the head, both eyes look backward up. [2] Turn the body to the right in the same way. (Fig. 10-17)

(7) Shrug the shoulders and turn backward

Starting form: The same as (5).

Movements: [1] Shrug the shoulders and turn backward. (Fig. 10-18) [2] Relax the shoulders and return to the original form.

(8) Draw the bow on both sides

Starting form: The same as (5).

Movements: [1] Bend the knees slightly, and turn the upper body to the left. At the same time, raise both forearms in front of the body, left hand above and right hand below, palm facing palm. When they are raised to chest level, pull the right hand backward and push the left hand upward to the left as if drawing a bow, eyes on the left hand. (Fig. 10-19) [2] After returning to the starting form, draw the bow on the right side.

(9) Lift the arms and raise the knees

Starting form: The same as (5).

Movements: [1] Lift the right arm sideways with the palm turned up, and at the same time raise the left knee. [2] Return to the starting form, and then lift the left arm and raise the right knee in the same way. (Fig. 10-20)

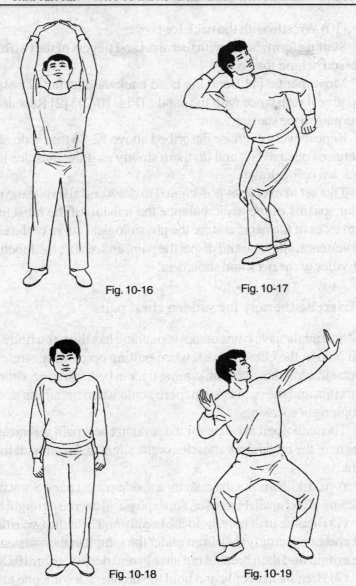

Fig. 10-16

Fig. 10-17

Fig. 10-18

Fig. 10-19

(10) Wrestle with the neck for power

Starting form: Stand with feet apart and fingers of the two hands crossed behind the neck.

Movements: [1] Bend the head backward as far as possible and give it resistance with the hands. (Fig. 10-21) [2] Repeat after returning to the starting form.

Repeat every exercise described above 12-16 times, do all the exercises once a day, and do them slowly as if the muscles in the neck are being drawn.

This set of exercises is designed to draw and alleviate the muscular spasms of the neck, balance the tension of the muscles on both sides of the neck, restore the physiological curve of the cervical vertebra, alleviate and dispel the pain, and restore the functional activities of the neck and shoulders.

4. Exercise therapy for sudden chest pain

You might have come across something like this: You find a sudden pain in the chest or back when putting on clothes, stretching yourself, scratching an itch, turning over in bed, standing, sitting or working, and the pain is even more acute when breathing deeply, coughing or speaking.

The pathological cause for the sudden chest pain is mainly the spasm of the respiratory muscles or the slight dislocation of the rib joint.

A pain-killer is not the cure for a sudden chest pain. Sometimes it has no effect at all. However, some physical exercises might help.

(1) Breathe in deeply, hold the breath, and beat the two sides of the chest with empty fists from under the armpit to the waist, or pat the armpit and then breathe out slowly and deeply. (Fig. 10-22)

(2) Breathe in deeply and hold the breath, ask someone to beat

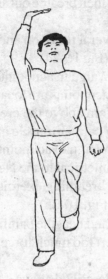

Fig. 10-20

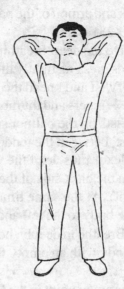

Fig. 10-21

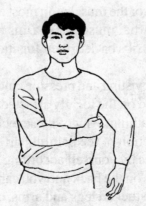

Fig. 10-22

201

the back and armpit of the painful side, and then breathe out slowly. (Fig. 10-23)

(3) Do the deep-breathing exercise several times on end, with the hands pressing tightly the painful part. (Fig 10-24)

(4) Twist and knead the Neiguan and Waiguan acupoints with the index fingers and thumb (the Neiguan acupoints are located on both wrists on the palmer side, about 6.6 cm above the crease of the wrist, between the tendons of the long palmar muscle and the radial flexor muscle of the wrist, and the Waiguan acupoint is located on the back side of the forearm, symmetrical to the Neiguan acupoint). At the same time, do the deep breathing exercise and twist the body to the left and to the right. (Fig. 10-25)

(5) Breathe in deeply, hold the breath, and beat the painful part of the body with an empty fist. Do not exert too much force. (Fig. 10-26)

A common point in the five exercises described above is "deep breathing." This is the gist of the treatment for the sudden chest pain, because deep breathing shortens but broadens the chest, thus increasing the tension of the muscles on most of the chest wall. This helps alleviate the partial muscular spasms and at the same time draws the joints of the ribs back to their functional positions to help relocate the joints.

Beating, patting, twisting and pressing, and massage are the different techniques used on the locally affected parts of the body on the basis of deep breathing. Any of these techniques can help restore the normal function of the painful part. You can also create some other techniques by yourself according to this principle. For example, if the pain is on the back and you cannot reach it, you can lie on a hard bed with tucked legs and arms, and roll to both sides several times. This also helps to kill the pain.

The cure for the sudden pain in the chest is simple. Some might

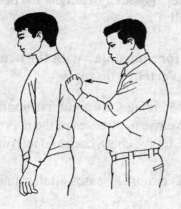

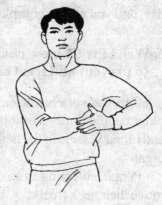

Fig. 10-23   Fig. 10-24

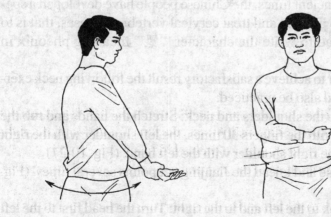

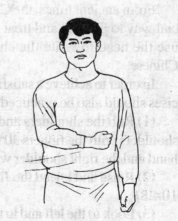

Fig. 10-25   Fig. 10-26

find it not immediately effective, but you will find the pain alleviated by 50-70 percent after a night's sleep. Another treatment the next day, and you will be completely well.

5. Write the Chinese character for "pheonix" with the head to prevent and treat cervical vertebra diseases

Cervical vertebra diseases, like lumbago, are common among older people. Strains or injuries give rise to diseases of the nerves and blood vessels in the head, neck, limbs, chest, back and internal organs.

People suffering from cervical vertebra diseases often cannot move their neck freely.

Western medicine usually treats such diseases by using gravitational force to reduce the pressure, while traditional Chinese medicine uses massage to help the patient invigorate the cervical vertebra.

From ancient times, the Chinese people have developed a special way to prevent and treat cervical vertebra diseases, that is to use the head to write the character " 鳳 " meaning pheonix in Chinese.

In order to achieve a satisfactory result the following neck exercises should also be practiced:

(1) Rub the shoulders and neck: Stretch the hands and rub the shoulders with the fingers 30 times, the left shoulder with the right hand and the right shoulder with the left hand. (Fig. 10-27)

(2) Raise and knead the Jianjing acupoints several times. (Fig. 10-28)

(3) Look to the left and to the right: Turn the head first to the left and look up backward. The movement should be slow and its range should be as large as possible. Then turn the head to the right and look up backward in the same way. (Figs. 10-29, 10-30)

(4) Stretch the neck backward: Lower the head slightly, and then stretch it slowly backward. When it is stretched backward to the utmost, shrink the neck muscle forcefully, and return to the original position. Repeat the exercise altogether 20 times. (Fig. 10-31)

(5) Turn the neck slowly: The movement should be slow and the range of movement should be gradually increased. Repeat this movement for 5-10 minutes. (Fig. 10-32)

This set of neck exercises is simple and easy to learn. It is different from the gravitational force method used in Western medicine, but has the equally satisfactory effect of improving the muscular power and stability of the neck.

These warming-up exercises are followed by the writing of the Chinese character "鳳," with the head. (Fig. 10-33)

It is written in this way:

Pivot the cervical vertebra, relax the head as much as possible, sway the neck, and write in the order and number of the strokes of the old character "鳳", stroke by stroke, in earnest way. When executing the movements, the range should be as large as possible to keep both the head and the neck fully engaged.

The stroke order is: First write the " 丿 " then "乙" then the horizontal stroke in the middle "一," then the character "鳥" for the bird written in this way: first " 丿 ," then " 丨 ," then "𠃌," then three horizontal strokes "一," followed by the stroke "𠃍," and finally the four dots from left to right "灬".

The reason the character "鳳" is used is perhaps because it implies good luck. This is because the pheonix is the king and queen of all birds in ancient legend. It has beautiful feathers, the male is called "feng" and the female is called "huang," and they are often used as a symbol of good luck. However, in this case it is perhaps because the character consists of complex strokes done in all directions, including horizontal, vertical, oblique, point and hook.

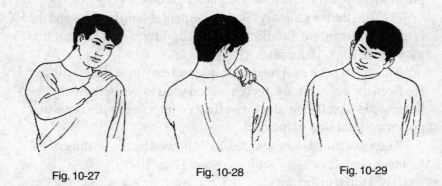

Fig. 10-27   Fig. 10-28   Fig. 10-29

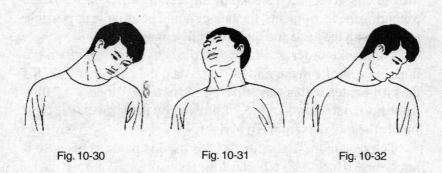

Fig. 10-30   Fig. 10-31   Fig. 10-32

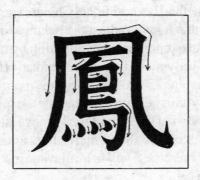

Fig. 10-33

This helps all parts of the neck to move in all directions so that the neck can be worked fully.

After finishing the neck exercises, use the head to write the character of pheonix three consecutive times. If you practise this twice or three times a day, you will surely get satisfactory results.

6. Rapping method to cure insomnia

People who do mental work are often troubled by insomnia because their overtaxed brain and excessive tension causes abnormalities in the central nervous system, which induces sleep. Insomnia often gives rise to dizziness, tinnitus and exhaustion. Serious cases can disrupt work and health.

Traditional Chinese medicine believes that insomnia is mainly caused by the functional imbalance of the heart and kidneys. The heart commands mental activities. When the heart is deficient in or loses its energy, this leads to amnesia and insomnia. The kidneys command the reproductive essence. If the reproductive essence is not sufficient, one is listless, sleeps less and is easily awakened.

The rapping method is a traditional Chinese exercise for the prevention of insomnia. It helps adjust the balance of the internal organs and abnormal excitement and inhibition by rapping the heart meridian of hand Shaoyin and the kidney meridian of the foot Shaoyin. The rhythmical rapping keeps stimulating the meridians of the heart and kidneys lightly, thus helping to invigorate the spleen, nourish the heart, replenish the vital essence of the kidneys and normalize the sleeping function. Practice shows that as long as one perseveres in doing the rapping exercise, it will help alleviate insomnia. Insomniacs might give it a try.

The rapping method is simple and easy to learn. It consists of four exercises, done in this way:

Exercise 1: Rap the legs

Sit with legs straight and use both palms to rap the inner side of the legs (equivalent to the transmission lines of the spleen, kidneys and liver meridians in the legs) and the outer side of the legs (equivalent to the transmission lines of the stomach and gallbladder meridians in the legs). Keep on rapping the two sides of the legs from the groin to the ankles alternately. (Fig. 10-34)

Exercise 2: Rap the waist

Sit with legs straight, put the hands on the two sides of the waist and rap the bulging muscles on the two sides of the waist with the backs of the hands. While rapping the waist, bend it forward and backward, but naturally and without much force. (Fig. 10-35)

Exercise 3: Rap the neck and shoulders

Sit and rap the left side of the neck with the finger tips of the right hand, starting from behind the ear, along the left side of the neck to the bulging part of the muscles of the left shoulder. Then rap the right side of the neck with the finger tips of the left hand, starting from behind the right ear, along the right side of the neck to the bulging part of the muscles of the right shoulder. Do this alternately. (Fig. 10-36)

Exercise 4: Rap the forearms

Sit with the left forearm and hand horizontally straight, palm facing up, then rap the side of the left forearm with the little finger (corresponding to the transmission line of the heart meridian in the forearm) from elbow to wrist with the palmar side of the fingers of the right hand. Then place the right forearm and hand horizontally, palm facing up, and rap the side of the right forearm with the little finger from elbow to wrist with the palmar side of the fingers of the left hand. Keep on rapping the forearms alternately. (Fig. 10-37)

Do the rapping exercise once every morning and evening. It takes about 15-20 minutes each time, that is, five minutes each for Exercises 1, 3 and 4, and three minutes for Exercise 2.

Points for attention:

[1] Relax the body, keep calm and quiet, breathe evenly and count the number of repititions silently.

[2] Rap with moderate force and rhythm. Do not exert too much force, and the sore, numb, swollen and warm sensations from the rapped parts should disappear within 15 minutes after rapping.

[3] Stretch the waist, legs, head and neck lightly after rapping.

[4] Do not do the exercises if the part or parts to be rapped suffer from skin disease, are swollen or infected.

In addition, in order to help insomniacs to fall asleep quickly, we would like to introduce you to a set of hypnotizing *qigong* exercises:

Hypnotizing exercises are simple and easy to do. You just lie on bed to do them. However, it should be the very last thing you do before going to bed. People suffering from chronic bronchitis and coughing with phlegm should first discharge all phlegm.

Lie on the back, legs straight, heels together and hands close by the thighs. All muscles of the body should be relaxed and the eyes

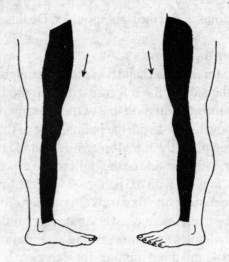

Fig. 10-34

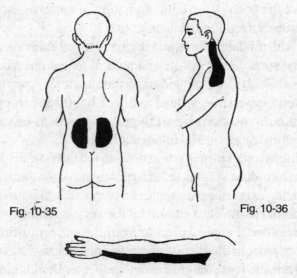

Fig. 10-35

Fig. 10-36

Fig. 11-37

closed. Breathe naturally. The most important thing is to free your mind of all distracting thoughts and induce your cerebrum into calm. Concentrate your mind on Dantian (about 5 cm below the navel). However, it is usually not easy to locate this point accurately, so instead you can use the simple and effective way of concentrating your mind on your big toe (either the left or the right, as you like).

In this way, you may fall asleep in a few minutes. If this does not work, maybe your cerebrum is not yet calm and quiet, and your mind is not yet concentrated on your big toe. If so, keep on doing the exercise, and you will get to sleep.

7. Exercise for treating pain in shoulder joints

Many people above 45 years of age often have pain in their shoulders because their joints are no longer as flexible, and sometimes they cannot raise their shoulders or stretch their arms upward. This is a common chronic disease among middle-aged people. It occurs most among people between the ages of 45 and 50, so it is commonly called "50-year-old shoulders" or "frozen shoulders," because the joints look as if they are frozen.

Traditional Chinese medicine holds that inflammation of the shoulder joints is mainly caused by wind-cold that attacks the shoulder joints.

The origin of the disease: When people reach 40 or 50 years old they usually become less active. Especially if they suffer from chronic diseases, and get little physical exercise. Because their shoulders and upper limbs are less active, the blood circulation becomes poor and the nutrients are insufficient, so the shoulder joints and their peripheral soft tissue begin to undergo retrogressive changes. Moreover, when people come to middle-age, their metabolism begins to slow down and signs of decline begin to occur throughout the body. The shoulder joints are, of course, no exception.

Sufferers often have pain in their shoulders accompanied by pressure. The pain is even worse at night and disturbs sleep. The pain is also very acute when the hands are raised or turned. This causes many difficulties in daily life.

There is no effective drug for this ailment. Here some methods are recommended to restore the function of the shoulder joints. Sufferers may do them all or in part:

(1) Swing arms: Stand with feet apart to shoulder width, swing the arms back and forth gently, and gradually increase the range of the movements. Do this exercise every morning and evening, 50-100 times. (Fig. 10-38)

(2) Scoop up: Stand with feet apart to shoulder width, bend the upper body forward and stretch the forearm on the side with pain downward as if scooping up something. Do this exercise 30-50 times every morning and evening. (Fig. 10-39)

(3) Draw circles: Stand with feet apart to shoulder width, keeping the body in position with the arms circling forward and backward, the range of movement going from small to large. Do this twice a day, 30-50 times each time. (Fig. 10-40)

(4) Touch the wall: Stand at the foot of the wall, put the hand of the affected side on the wall, and touch it from below upward to the highest point, and then put the hand down. Repeat this 20-30 times each time. (Fig. 10-41)

(5) Shrug the shoulders: Sit or stand. Bend the elbow joints to an angle of 90 degrees, and shrug the shoulders, first weakly and then powerfully. Do this twice a day, 50-100 times each time. (Fig. 10-42)

(6) Touch the highest: Use a tree branch or hang something in the room as a marker. Try your best to touch it with the hand on the affected side, and gradually increase the height. Do this twice a day,

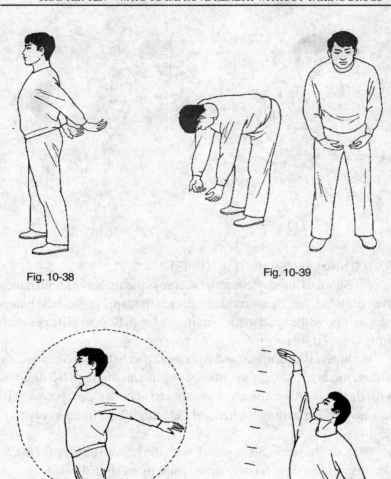

Fig. 10-38

Fig. 10-39

Fig. 10-40

Fig. 10-41

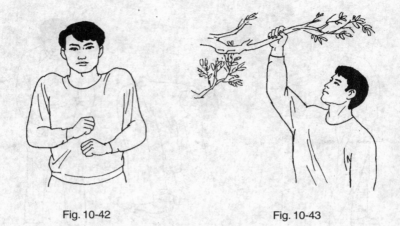

Fig. 10-42   Fig. 10-43

50-100 times each time. (Fig. 10-43)

(7) Shoot to the sky: Stand or sit, cross the fingers of both hands over the head, and then gradually stretch the arms to raise the hands upward above the head to the maximum limit. Repeat 30 times each time. (Fig. 10-44)

(8) Spread the arms: Stand with feet apart to the shoulder width, stretch the arms to the two sides, forming an angle of 90 degrees with the body. After the arms are spread at both sides, pause 5-10 seconds before putting them down. Do this 30-50 times every day. (Fig 10-45)

(9) Rub the neck: Sit or stand, with the hands rubbing the neck. Do this twice a day, 50-100 times each time. (Fig. 10-46)

8. Walking backward exercise for lumbago

Functional lumbago is usually referred to as "strain of the lumbar muscles," and mostly occurs among middle-aged and older people. It can last a long time with severe pain. This can be treated with

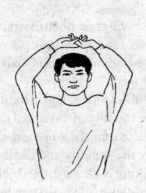

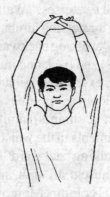

Fig. 10-44

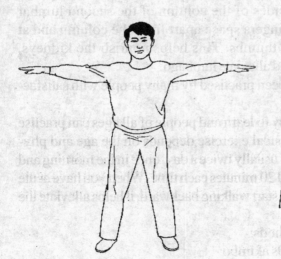

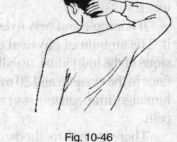

Fig. 10-46

Fig. 10-45

physical exercises. "Walking backward" is an effective exercise therapy for treating lumbago.

The "walking backward" exercise will strengthen the muscles in the waist and back and increase muscle strength.

This exercise originates from the traditional Taiji Quan movement known as "monkey steps backward."

Lumbar strain is mainly due to insufficient strength of the muscles and ligaments in the waist, with poor stability of the spinal column. The "walking backward" exercise helps train the waist muscles, increase muscle strength, and improve the stability and flexibility of the spinal column. Moreover, in walking backward, the rhythmical contraction and relaxation of the muscles in the waist can improve the blood circulation and tissue metabolism. When walking backward, it is also necessary to massage the Shenshu acupoints (located on the two sides of the column of the second lumbar vertebra, about two fingers space apart from the column and at navel level) with the thumbs. This helps nourish the kidneys, strengthen the waist and alleviate lumbago.

This exercise has been practised by many people with satisfactory results.

It is simple and easy to learn and people of all ages can practise it. The amount of physical exercise depends on the age and physique of the individual, usually twice a day, once in the morning and once in the evening and 20 minutes each time. When you have acute lumbago, immediately start walking backward, it helps alleviate the pain.

There are two methods:

(1) Walk with hands akimbo:

Starting form: Stand erect, chest out, head up, eyes front, hands akimbo with the thumbs pressing the Shenshu acupoints.

Description: Begin with the left leg. Raise the left thigh backward as much as possible and step backward. Shift the body weight backward, land the foot first with the ball and then the sole. Shift the body weight to the left leg and change to the right leg. Walk this way with the feet moving backward alternately. Press the Shenshu points with both thumbs once with each step. Move 40 steps per minute, and at least 600 steps in 20 minutes.

(2) Walk with arms swinging:

Starting form: Stand erect, chest out, head up, eyes front and arms down.

Description: The leg movements are the same as in (1). Swing the arms while walking backward.

Essential points: Keep the chest out and raise the thighs backward as much as possible.

Points for attention: Choose either way or use both ways alternately. The ground must be flat with no obstacles. Sufferers from tuberculosis or tumors should not do this exercise. Those with acute pain in the waist should first find out the cause, and can do the exercise if it is a functional condition. Moreover, this exercise also helps prevent humpback because it increases the physical exertion backward and stretches the trunk, thus adjusting the imbalance of the trunk bending forward or backward.

9. Patting method for treating pain in the shoulder and waist

Pain in the shoulder and waist mostly originates with muscle spasms, inflammation and tissue contraction. Traditional Chinese medicine believes that in most cases this is because external wind-cold causes partial stasis of the vital energy and blood, and obstruction of some meridians.

In his book *The Thousand Golden Formulae*, Sun Simiao of the Tang Dynasty wrote: "If the hands feel cold, pat from top to bottom until they feel warm," and "if the feet feel cold, pat until they feel warm." In other words, use massage to treat it.

In traditional Chinese medicine it is also said that "the blood flows when it is warm" and "warm it when it is cold." In other words, blood circulation is conditioned by warm temperature, and diseases due to cold should be treated by warm methods.

The four patting exercises for treating shoulder and waist pain worked out on the basis of this theory have a satisfactory curative effect.

The exercises are as follows:

(1) Pat the arms:

Starting form: Stand naturally with feet apart.

Description: Raise one arm horizontally forward (not necessarily straight), and pat the shoulder, arm, wrist and hand with the other hand, and pat back and forth the three lines of the front, middle and rear parts of the shoulder and arm. Pat the arms with the left and right hands alternately. (Fig. 10-47)

Number of times: Pat 12-24 times on each side.

Effect: It promotes blood circulation and the flow of vital energy, removes obstruction in the collaterals in the shoulders and arms, relaxes the joints and muscles, and alleviates the pain.

(2) Stroke the shoulders and back:

Starting form: Stand with feet apart.

Description: Pat the left shoulder with the right palm and stroke the back on the right side with the back of the left hand. Pat the right shoulder with the left palm and stroke the back on the left side with the back of the right hand. Pat and stroke alternately. (Fig. 10-48)

Number of times: Repeat 12-24 times on each side.

Effect: It relaxes the shoulders and back, removes the spasm, removes the obstruction in the channels and collaterals of the meridian system, and prevents and treats soreness and pain.

218

(3) Pat and knock the Shenshu acupoints

Starting form: Stand with feet apart.

Description: Pat and knock the Shenshu acupoints with the palms, the back of both hands and the back of the fists in rotation. (Fig. 10-49)

Number of times: Repeat 12-24 times on each side.

Effect: It strengthens the kidneys to nourish seminal reproduction, promotes blood circulation, removes numbness and prevents lumbago.

(4) Shake the waist and swing the arms

Starting form: Stand with feet apart.

Description: Relax the body and use the hands to drive the arms. Use the arms to drive the waist and swing them to the left and right to beat the waist (mainly pat the waist with the back of the hands). (Fig. 10-50)

Number of times: Repeat 12-24 times on each side.

Effect: It relaxes the sacrum and buttocks, invigorates the meridian system, replenishes the kidneys, cures diseases and prolongs life.

Points for attention:

[1] When patting or stroking, the force exerted must be increased gradually. It is better to do it slowly, and take it easy.

[2] The exercise time and number of times for practice differ from person to person. The number of times is not compulsory. Beat to the point that the beaten part feels warm. Usually, 2-4 times a day, half an hour before or after meals, and 20 minutes each time.

[3] The amount of physical exercise should be well-controlled. "Increase it when you feel sore, reduce it when you have a pain, and stop it when you feel numb." If you have sore muscles and feel swollen when raising the hands, increase the amount of exercise and continue the practice. If you have partial pain and the pain develops

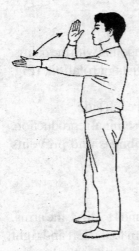

Fig. 11-47

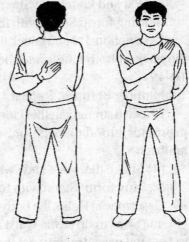

Fig. 11-48

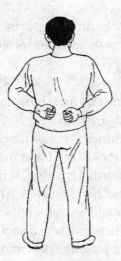

Fig. 10-49

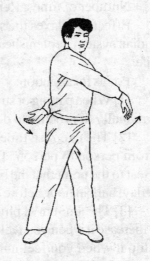

Fig. 10-50

gradually, this shows that a certain muscle or tendon has a hidden inflammation and the amount of exercise should be reduced to avoid aggravating the inflammation. If you find certain parts numb, it is a sign that a certain nerve is being pressed and the practice method is not correct. You must stop immediately, find the cause, and continue when the condition is corrected.

[4] Take off your outer garments before practice. If it is very cold, take off the garment after you warm up with one or two exercises. When the exercises are finished, put the garments on again to avoid wind. If your underwear becomes wet after sweating, change to dry and clean clothes.

Contraindications:

[1] Stop practising if you have acute inflammation locally, high fever or bleeding.

[2] Do not practise if you cannot control your emotions because it is very difficult for you to execute the movements accurately and it is easy to injure yourself if you are emotionally upset.

The patting exercises are specially suitable for older and physically weak people and sufferers from pain in the loins, back, shoulders and arms. Although the movements are few, as long as you persevere in doing them, you will achieve noticeable results.

10. Rubbing abdomen to treat gastric and intestinal diseases

The abdomen rubbing exercise is also called the method of curing diseases and prolonging life. It is a common technique used for health preservation among the Chinese, and has been widely practised since the Qing Dynasty.

This exercise is intended mainly to accelerate blood circulation in the abdomen and stimulate the nerve receptors on the membranes of the stomach and intestines by rubbing certain acupoints and affected parts and massaging and drawing the internal organs directly to cause the excitation of the vagus nerve under the regulation of the central nervous system, thus promoting the contraction of the smooth muscles in the stomach and intestines and strengthening their peristalsis. At the same time, it also helps promote the secretion of gastric juice, bile, pancreatic juice and small intestinal juice, improve the digestion and absorption of food by the stomach and intestines, and increase the liver's metabolism of sugar, protein and fats.

It helps cure certain gastric and intestinal diseases, including gastric ulcer, duodenal ulcer, chronic gastritis, gastric and intestinal neurosis, inflammation of the colon and habitual constipation.

(1) Starting form:

Sit or lie on your back. If sitting, keep the upper part of the body upright, feet on the ground and apart to a little wider than shoulder width. If lying, bend the knees slightly, feet slightly apart and heels on the bed. In winter, or when it is otherwise cold, lie on the bed with a quilt on, or sit under the quilt with clothes on.

(2) Methods:

[1] Rub Zhongwan: Put the cushions of the three middle fingers of the right hand on the pit of the stomach and press the three middle fingers of the left hand on them. Exert force with both hands and press-rub gently around the Zhongwan point (the midpoint on the anterior midline of the upper abdomen between the joint of the ribs and the navel, Fig. 10-51) clockwise 36 times. (Fig. 10-52)

[2] Rub the navel: Massage gently the parts around the navel 18 circles clockwise, with the cushions of the three middle fingers of the right hand and the left hand fingers on top of the right, starting from the left side of the navel. Then change to the left hand, start from the right side of the navel and rub gently around the navel counterclockwise 18 times.

[3] Rub the Qihai and Guanyuan acupoints (Fig. 10-51): Turn-

rub around with the cushions of the three middle fingers of the right hand and the left hand fingers on top of the right hand, starting from the Qihai acupoint downward to the lower-left, past the Guanyuan acupoint, upward to the upper-right and back to Qihai. Massage this way 18 times. Then change to the left hand and turn-rub gently in the opposite direction 18 times.

[4] Push the Ren channel (Fig. 10-53): Push gently with the cushions of the three middle fingers of one hand (the three middle fingers of the other hand on top of them) from the pit of the stomach, along the midline of the abdomen down to the joint of the pubic bones. Move the three middle fingers of the hands separately outward, and push-rub along the fossa iliaca upward along the line under the nipples to the rib-bows, then toward the pit of the stomach, and finally back to the pit of the stomach with the three middle fingers of one hand on top of the other three middle fingers. This counts as one circle. Repeat this 36 times. Women do this exercise by using the turn-rubbing method.

[5] Rub the entire abdomen (Fig. 10-54): Keep the left hand akimbo with the thumb in front (left hand in free position when lying), push and rub gently from the lower right of the lower abdomen (the right fossa iliaca) with the right palm, past the right hypochondrium (above the breastline), the left hypochondrium to the left side of the lower abdomen the left fossa iliaca, and finally back to the lower-right of the lower abdomen. This counts as a circle. Do this 18 times. And then change to the left palm and go along the same route in the opposite direction 18 times.

[6] Point-press and rock: Use these techniques to assist the above-described techniques to achieve an even better result.

Point-press: Use two or three middle fingers of one hand to press the Zhongwan, Guanyuan and Qihai acupoints. Push the fingers downward and then lift them up slowly. This is one repitition.

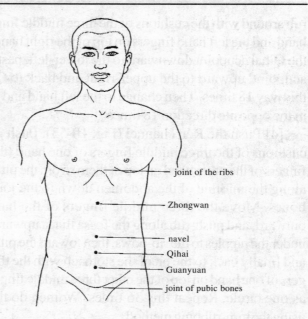

- joint of the ribs
- Zhongwan
- navel
- Qihai
- Guanyuan
- joint of pubic bones

Fig. 10-51

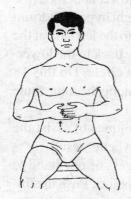

Fig. 10-52

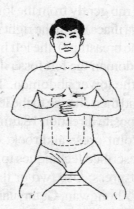

Fig. 10-53

Press each acupoint 5-7 times.

Push-press: Use the base of the palm to push and press the loins. Before pressing, put the hands on the loins, finger tips ahead, and the thumbs tightly against the lower edge of the rib-bows. When push pressing inward and forward energetically with the palm bases, the abdomen bulges, and when loosening the palm bases, the abdomen withdraws to the original position. This is one repitition. Do this 9 times in a row. (Fig. 10-55)

Rock: Place the hands to the knees and sit with legs crossed, rock the upper body clockwise 9 times and then counterclockwise 9 times, with the rocking range increased gradually. (Fig. 10-56)

(3) Number of times:

Press-rub the abdomen two or three times a day, in the morning and in the evening. The number of times for each movement depends on your own physical condition. When disease occurs, greatly increase the number of times. If you have abdominal pain, you can increase it to several dozen or even several hundred times until the

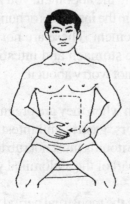

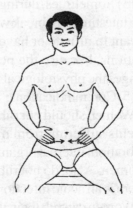

Fig. 10-54   Fig. 10-55

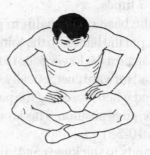

Fig. 10-56

signs of the illness are eased or gone. In short, you should feel soothed, relaxed and free from fatigue after rubbing and pressing.

(4) Points for attention:

[1] Concentrate the mind, focus the attention and breathe naturally.

[2] The movements should be gentle, slow and continuous. Do not exert too much force in order to avoid injuring the internal organs.

[3] Sometimes, during or after rubbing the abdomen, you may have intestinal gas, break wind, feel warm in the intestines or hungry, or want to urinate or have a bowel movement. These are normal reactions, because the peristalsis of the stomach and intestines changes the physiological functions. Do not worry about it.

(5) Contraindications:

Women should not rub their abdomen when they are pregnant. Patients suffering from malignant tumors, gastric and intestinal perforation, internal organ bleeding or peritonitis must not rub their abdomen. Also, do not rub the affected part of the abdominal wall if there is an acute infection.

Women can rub their abdomen during the menstrual period, but they should be sure not to catch cold. It is not good to rub the abdomen when you are too hungry or too full. If you want to urinate or have a bowel movement, please do so before rubbing.

11. "Sleep-sit-stand" exercises for sciatica

Deep in the muscles of the buttocks, on each side, lies the sciatic nerve, starting from the sacrum of the spinal cord, running down along the thighs, and branching out gradually through the shanks to the muscles and skin of the soles of the feet. This is an important nerve, controlling the movement and feeling of the legs. Sciatica is a common and frequently occurring disease affecting this nerve.

Once the sciatic nerve is inflamed or pressed by neighboring bones, ligaments, tumors, inflammation of the muscles, and especially the protrusion of the intervertebral disc, there is pain in this nerve. In an acute condition, the pain extends from the lumbar area to the feet, making it difficult to walk. Even if it becomes chronic, there is always hidden pain as if something is drawing it, and movement of the legs and feet is difficult.

If you have sciatica, you should first discover the cause. If it is caused by pathological changes that constrict the nerve, this problem must be solved. If it is an inflammation of the sciatic nerve itself, you should lie in bed and rest during the acute period and treat it with painkillers, acupuncture or massage. If it is chronic, please do the exercise described in the following passages.

Traditional Chinese medicine believes that the limbs must move about to reduce strain. Therefore, once you are afflicted with sciatica, you should continue to move the lower limbs so the condition does not become aggravated.

Because the pain during the chronic period is often related to adhesion around the nerve, the "sleep-sit-stand" method is called for so the sciatic nerve has a chance to recover. Repeated practice helps to dissolve the adhesion and relieve the pain.

The method is described as follows:

Sleep: Lie on the bed on your back with legs bent, stretch the legs by rotation with the feet on the bed, and then raise the legs upward by rotation. Usually, the leg on the healthy side can be raised from the bed at a 90 degree angle, and the leg on the affected side to a 45 degree at first, with the angle gradually increased after practice. (Fig. 10-57)

Sit: Sit on the bedside or in a chair with legs straight, heels on the ground, toes up, and hands on the thighs. Bend the body forward gradually and push the hands toward the feet. At first, the hands cannot reach far, but they will be able to reach the insteps and toes after repeated practice. (Fig. 10-58)

Stand: Stand upright with hands akimbo. First raise the legs forward by rotation, knees straight, and then stand with the feet as far apart as possible, and bend the knees by rotation. Squat down like a bow so that the straight leg is straightened and drawn with a pulling force. (Fig. 10-59)

Sufferers of sciatica should also do some running, physical exercise or play ball games as much as possible, all beneficial to the recovery of health.

12. Point-pressing for fainting, lumbago and seminal emission

Point-pressing is a therapy in which fingers replace needles to press certain acupoints for the treatment of some diseases. If used properly, it often produces an instant curative effect.

The point-pressing therapy described here is good for the treatment of headache, fainting, acute lumbar sprain, angina pectoris and seminal emission.

(1) Press the temples to treat headache

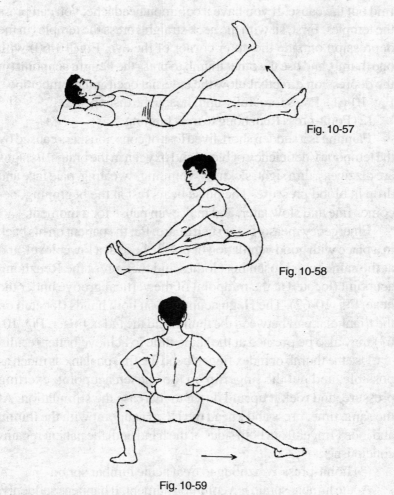

Fig. 10-57

Fig. 10-58

Fig. 10-59

There are many factors for the headache. You should first of all find out the cause. If you have a common headache, you can press the temples. First, sit with the neck straight, press the temple (in the depression outside the outer corner of the eye, Fig. 10-60) with one thumb, and use the other thumb to press the Fengfu acupoint (in the depression directly below the external occipital protuberance, Fig. 10-61). Press forcefully until headache disappears.

(2) Point-press Renzhong to treat fainting

Fainting is a sudden short-lived loss of consciousness caused by the temporary deficiency of blood and oxygen in the brains. Its signs are dizziness, dim sight, sickness, vomiting, sweating, pale face and drop in blood pressure. The pulse beats fast at the beginning, becomes fine and slow later, and may even pause for a moment.

Emergency measures for such a case: Put the patient on his back in a place with good ventilation or put the head at a lower level, and at the same time loosen his clothes and then press the Renzhong acupoint (located at the midpoint of the vertical groove under the nose, Fig. 10-62). The Hegu acupoints on both hands (located on the triangular part between the thumb and the index finger, Fig. 10-63) may also be pressed at the same time to achieve better result.

Use the thumb or index finger, bend the first phalanx as much as possible, and put the fingertip on the chosen acupoint, exerting pressure, and rock it up and down to increase the stimulation. At the same time, press and knead the Hegu acupoint with the thumb and index finger from both sides of the hand until the patient regains conciousness.

(3) Point-press Weizhong to treat acute lumbar sprain

Acute lumbar sprain is a common ailment. It happens suddenly, in most cases during physical activity, sometimes when bending or turning the body abruptly. Symptoms are acute lumbar pain and inability to exert force, "stiff waist" with difficulty walking or an in-

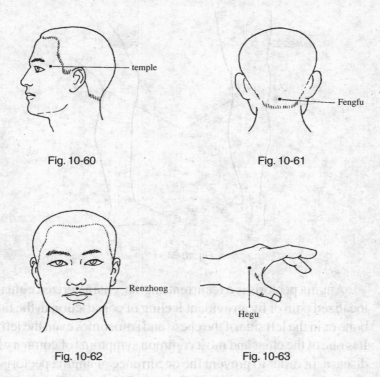

Fig. 10-60   Fig. 10-61

Fig. 10-62   Fig. 10-63

ability to walk. Sometimes the waist cannot move at all. If it does, it causes an acute pain like an electric shock. Pressing the Weizhong acupoints will produce a good curative effect.

Put the patient face-down, legs straight. The Weizhong acupoints are located on both legs, at the midpoint of the popliteal crease in the depression of the knees. (Fig. 10-64) Use the tip of the right thumb (with the nail cut) to press at Weizhong forcefully and turn in a circle. It is better to have the patient cry aloud. Point-press the point twice on end and the lumbar pain disappears.

(4) Point-press the Neiguan acupoints to treat angina pectoris

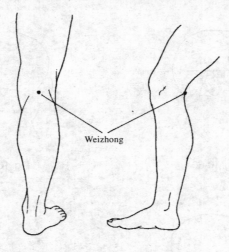

Fig. 10-64

Angina pectoris is a recurrent angina, characterized either by a localized pain or by an evident feeling of constriction in the breast-bone or in the left side of the chest, and sometimes even the left arm. It is one of the chief and most common symptoms of coronary heart disease. In order to prevent the occurrence of angina pectoris, one may take nitroglycerine and Guanxin Suhe pills (Storax Pills for Coronary Heart Disease) orally or receive the cupping therapy on the back. They both have very good preventive and curative effects. However, if you have not taken preventive measures in advance, and you have a sudden attack of angina pectoris, point-press force-fully the Neiguan acupoint (located on the palmar side of the forearm, 6.6 cm above the crease of the wrist) with the nail of your right thumb until the pain disappears. You can also supplement this by pressing the Hegu acupoint.

(5) Point-press Huiyin to treat seminal emission

Seminal emission includes nocturnal emission and spermatorrhea. In the former case, the semen is involuntarily discharged in dreams while in the latter case, it happens without dreams. People affected by emission are often listless and dizzy, and suffer from tinnitus, bad memory, weariness, chronic pain in the loins and legs, palpitations and shortness of breath. It not only affects work and study, but also affects the health of the mind and body.

An effective treatment for emission is point-pressing the Huiyin acupoint: Press the Huiyin point between the anus and the genitals with the middle finger of the right hand (Fig. 10-66) to produce mixed sensation of numbness, distention and soreness. Press it for 1-2 minutes each time. Press it in a lying position, legs bent and apart, so that the point is fully exposed to the pressure.

The five methods described above are unique skills and treasures of traditional Chinese medicine. Before the disease occurs, the patient can do it by himself to prevent the occurrence of the disease. If the disease occurs, someone else has to help the patient do it. If used properly, it will cure the illness instantly. The methods are simple, but the curative effects are satisfactory.

13. "Anus-raising" exercise for treating hemorrhoids

A common Chinese saying goes: "Nine out of ten men have hemorrhoids." Although this is not completely correct, it shows that hemorrhoids is one of the most common chronic diseases and the rate of occurrence is as high as 60-70 percent.

During the late stages of hemorrhoids, there are often complications such as the prolapse of the anus, anemia, anal fistula, and abscess.

The "anus-raising" exercise described here is a simple, easy-to-learn and practical method of preventing and curing hemorrhoids.

Contraction of the anus was in fact introduced in ancient times in

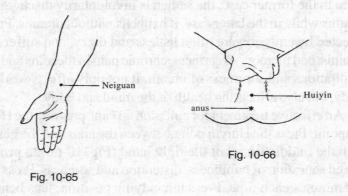

Fig. 10-65

Fig. 10-66

China. In his book *Zhen Zhong Fang* (*Prescriptions in the Pillow,*) Sun Simiao, a famous Tang Dynasty physician, wrote about the contraction of the anus.

Qigong practitioners also advocate that "Huiyin (perineum) under the crotch should be well protected."

The occurrence of hemorrhoids is related to difficulty in the flow back of the blood in the veins. The return of the blood in the veins to the heart depends mainly on the contraction and relaxation of the muscles. Long-time sitting without movement, physical weakness, and the accumulation of fats in the abdomen all make the muscles around the rectum and anus less powerful, thus affecting the backflow of the blood in the veins and resulting in the expansion of the veins and blood stasis at the lower end of the rectum, and hemorrhoids.

If you do the "anus-raising" exercise, it helps to work up the muscles around the anus and increase their power, thus preventing the expansion of the veins. Assisted by breathing exercises, it can also improve the function of the cardiovascular system, accelerate the backflow of the blood in the veins, reduce blood pressure, and remove blood stasis in the rectum and anus. Moreover, it also stimulates the peristalsis of the intestines and sases constipation. Therefore, the "anus-raising" exercise helps improve the blood circulation in the peripheral tissues of the anus so that hemorrhoids can be prevented.

There is a pithy formula for the exercise: "Inhale, lick, raise and hold." Inhale means breathing in, lick means licking the upper jaw, raise means contracting the anus, and hold means holding the breath. These movements must be executed simultaneously.

It should be done like this: Relax the entire body, press the buttocks and thighs tightly against each other, draw in a breath with the tongue licking the upper jaw, and at the same time, raise the anus upward as if holding back a bowel movement. Hold the breath for a moment after raising the anus, then breathe out and relax the whole body.

This exercise is simple, and can be done any time and any place you wish, sitting, lying down, or standing. Generally, this should be done twice a day, once in the morning and once in the evening.

Points for attention:

[1] This exercise is good for internal hemorrhoids, external hemorrhoids, prolapse of the anus and anal fistula. However, if there is an acute anal fissure, inflammation of piles, abscess around the anus, prolapse of the anus, or acute inflammation, do the exercise only after they are cured.

[2] You must have perseverance, and do the exercise everyday without interruption.

[3] Eat less pungent foods

[4] Do not sit too long during a bowel movement, and do not read.

[5] Take care to eliminate all factors that may cause hemorrhoids, and prevent constipation in particular.

[6] Take some other supplementary measures while doing the

"anus-raising" exercise such as washing the anus with warm water after bowel movements or before sleep, hot compression for the anus, and massaging the muscles around the anus to promote blood circulation. The curative effect is still better if you also do *qigong* exercises.

14. Waist-turning exercise—a good cure for constipation

Chronic constipation is a common malady. It occurs mostly among middle-aged and elderly people, the physically weak, people with chronic diseases and those recovering from surgery. There are many causes of habitual constipation such as longtime sitting, lack of physical exercise or work, an irregular life, irregular bowel movements, not eating enough fiber-rich foods, and drinking too little. The most important factor is lack of physical exercise. This weakens the contracting power of the intestinal, abdominal, and anal muscles, reduces the strength of the peristalsis of the intestinal canal, keeps the food in the intestines too long with too much waterabsorbed, thus drying and hardening the stool.

Here, we would like to recommend a set of waist-turning exercises —a good cure for chronic constipation widely practised among Chinese people. It is easy to learn and has a good curative effect.

The waist-turning exercises are intended to strengthen the muscular power of the abdominal wall and increase the secretion of the intestinal juice by training the muscles around the waist, in the abdomen, and in the pelvic cavity, thus promoting the peristalsis of the stomach and intestines so that the movement of the intestinal canal becomes normal and makes it easier to discharge excrement. Moreover, the exercises also help regulate nerve reaction, improve the regulation of the gastric and intestinal activities by the nervous system, and cure functional disorders of the intestines such as constipation and diarrhea.

The waist-turning exercises are done this way:

Starting form: Stand with feet apart and toes obliquely outward in the shape of V, slightly wider than shoulder width. Keep the upper body upright, hands akimbo, and knees slightly bent. (Fig. 10- 67)

Description: Turn the waist and abdomen with the navel as the pivot in the following directions:

[1] Turn to the left→ forward→ right→ backward, clockwise horizontally. (Fig. 10-68)

[2] Turn to the right→ forward→ left→ backward, counter-clockwise horizontally. (Fig. 10-69)

[3] Turn to the left→ downward→ right→ upward, vertically from left to right like a turning wheel. (Fig. 10-70)

[4] Turn to the right→ downward→ left→ upward, vertically from right to left like a turning wheel. (Fig. 10-71)

Points for attention:

[1] The main stress should be on the waist and abdomen, not on the shoulders or knees. Keep the shoulders and knees still or moving slightly. At the beginning, it is difficult to avoid turning the upper body, but you should gradually grasp the gist of it and turn the waist and abdomen only. Keep both the upper body and the legs almost still.

[2] One turn is counted as one repitition. Practise 1-3 sessions a day. The amount of physical exertion depends on your physical condition and the severity of the problem. Proceed step by step, and increase the amount of exertion gradually. Generally, turn 20 times every session at the beginning, and gradually increase to around 200 times. The time can be increased gradually from 30 seconds a session to 10 minutes a session.

[3] If you persevere in doing the first two of these four exercises for a few months, it will prove effective in curing constipation. If you can do all four exercises persistently, it will not only help to cure

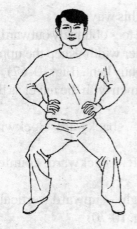

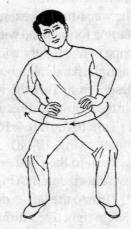

Fig. 10-67

Fig. 10-68

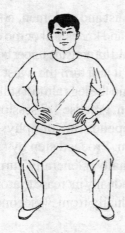

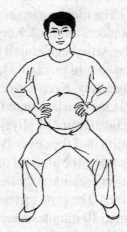

Fig. 10-69

Fig. 10-70

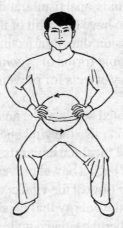

Fig. 10-71

chronic constipation and diarrhea, but will also strengthen the waist and the kidneys.

[4] It is appropriate to do the exercises in the early morning, before sleep or between meals. It is not good to do them right after eating or when you are too hungry. Eat foods rich in fiber and get into the habit of having bowel movements at regular times.

[5] If you have a fever, gastric or intestinal tumors, or bleeding stools, you should not do this exercise. And stop doing the exercise during a period of chronic disease or when you are dizzy or anemic.

[6] The results will be even better if you do self-massage on the abdomen in addition to the waist-turning exercises.

15. *Qigong* therapy for emission, hemorrhoids, and urinary incontinence

Elderly and physically weak people often suffer from

spermatorrhea, hemorrhoids, anal fistula, and urinary incontinence. Some young people who have the habit of masturbation may also suffer from frequent emission, directly affecting the health of the body and mind. The four simple forms of *qigong* exercises described here produce satisfactory effects for preventing and curing these diseases.

The perineum is located between the anus and the genitals. By raising the perineum, you raise the vital energy lightly so that the anus, the urethra and the local muscular tissues in this region are contracted, as if holding back a bowel movement. Its purpose is to use the mind to guide the flow of the vital energy so that the energy which flows down and the energy that is raised up communicate with each other to strengthen the kidneys and arrest seminal emission. From the viewpoint of modern medical science, raising the perineum consciously from time to time helps to improve the blood circulation and the nutrition of the peripheral tissues of the perineum and improve the relaxing and contracting functions and restricting ability of the sphincters of the anus and bladder, as well as the muscular tissues of the genitals. Therefore, it is beneficial for the prevention and treatment of emission, spermatorrhea, inpotence, premature ejaculation, hemorrhoids, anal fistula, prolapse of the anus, and urinary incontinence.

This *qigong* therapy consists of four exercises:

(1) Lying on the back (Fig. 10-72)

[1] Lie on the back, head on a slightly raised pillow, feet level, and arms and hands naturally by the sides.

[2] Lick the tongue against the upper jaw, the eyes and lips slightly closed, with high concentration free from distracting thoughts, and mind focused on Dantian. When saliva is secreted automatically in the mouth, draw in a fresh breath through the nose, use the mind to guide the flow of *qi* (vital energy) and then raise the perineum

lightly. At the same time, clench the teeth tightly, clench the fists energetically, bend the toes downward and forward energetically, and hold the breadth for 3-5 seconds. Then put the tongue down lightly, breathe out slowly, and relax the whole body.

[3] Lick the tongue against the upper jaw again, continue to do the same movements described above, and repeat all movements in the same way for 5-10 minutes each time, three times a day, in the morning, at noon and in the evening.

The lying-on-the-back exercise is good for preventing and treating emission, spermatorrhea, impotence, premature ejaculation and urinary incontinence.

(2) Slow walking (Fig. 10-73)

[1] Walk in slow steps as if taking a slow stroll, with high concentration, free from distracting thoughts, lips slightly closed with tongue licking the upper jaw, clench the upper and lower teeth

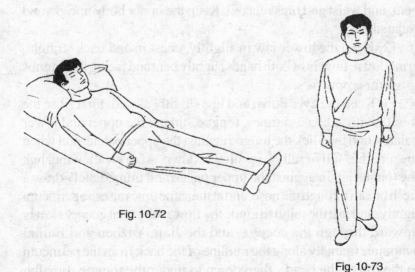

Fig. 10-72

Fig. 10-73

slightly, and with the mind focused on Dantian.

[2] Keep the hands down naturally, fingers slightly bent and facing the thumb to form semi-empty fists, toes of both feet hooking down as if grabbing the ground. Take a slow walk and raise the perineum lightly.

[3] After strolling slowly for 3-5 minutes, relax the perineum slowly, and take another slow walk for 1-2 minutes. Then continue to repeat the above movements. Do this exercise for about half an hour each time, after getting up in the morning and before going to bed in the evening.

These slow-walking and perineum-raising exercises help prevent and cure hemorrhoids, anal fistula, prolapse of the anus and urinary incontinence.

(3) Standing stake (Fig. 10-74)

[1] Stand with legs naturally apart, feet parallel to each other at shoulder width, toes of both feet grabbing the ground, knees slightly bent, and waist and hips relaxed. Keep the upper body upright and squat silghtly.

[2] Keep the lower jaw in slightly, chest in and back straight, arms down, fingers of both hands slightly bent and facing the thumbs in a semi-empty fists.

[3] Keep the eyes down and lips slightly closed. First rinse the mouth with saliva 3-5 times, tongue stirring the upper and lower palates, and then lick the tongue against the upper palate, and when the mouth is full of saliva, swallow it down. After swallowing, lick the tongue again against the upper palate and immediately draw a fresh breath through the nose, and at the same time raise the perineum lightly, and use the mind to guide the flow of the vital energy slowly upward through the coccyx, and the Jiaji, Yuzhen and Baihui acupoints (namely along the midline of the back from the perineum to the top of the head), then down to under the tongue. Finally,

breathe out slowly and relax the perineum. Repeat these movements 20 times, and then put the right hand on top of the left to press Dantian with the mind focused on it for a while, and take 30-50 slow steps.

This exercise should be done twice a day, once in the morning and once in the evening. It is good for treating all the conditions mentioned above.

(4) Sitting (Fig. 10-75)

Sit in a chair or on a square stool, thighs parallel to the ground. Keep the upper body upright, hands in semi-fists placed on the knees. Keep the eyes down and lips lightly closed. Lick the tongue against the upper palate. Other movements are the same as those in the Standing Stake. After finishing the exercise, rise and take 30-50 slow steps.

This exercise should also be done once in the morning and once

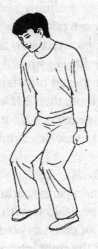

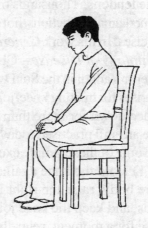

Fig. 10-74   Fig. 10-75

in the evening. Add a session at noon if you wish, as it is good for treating all the conditions mentioned above.

16. Knee-bending exercises for sore knees

The knee joint is one of the joints carrying a large load in bearing the body's weight, and in all activities. Walking, moving, sitting, lying, running and jumping are all impossible without it. Therefore, the knee joint is often subject to injury. Excessive activity may cause strain, while unexpected twists and falls can result in sprains or contusions. And remaining too long in cold and damp places may cause rheumatism in the legs. All these conditions will make it difficult for the knee joint to move about, bend, and stretch.

Traditional Chinese medicine believes that the knee joint is the meeting place for the tendons in the lower limbs. If the knee joint cannot bend and extend freely, you must bend your body or have some support when walking. This is a sign of the declining function of the tendons. Thousands of years ago, Chinese people began to use medicinal decoctions, hot compression, acupuncture and Daoyin exercises. In his work *General Treatise on the Etiology and Symptomatology of Diseases*, Chao Yuanfang, imperial physician to emperor Yangdi in the Sui Dynasty, collected more than 20 Daoyin exercises for treating knee-joint diseases. These methods have been handed down for more than 1,000 years, and exercises similar to these are still practised today.

Some of these simple exercises are as follows:

(1) Hold the knee against the chest: Stand upright, relax the entire body, raise the right leg, bend the knee, hold it with both hands, and keep the knee joint as close to your chest as possible. Pause for a moment, relax the hands, and put the right leg back to its original position. Then raise the left leg, and execute the move-

ments in the same way as the right leg. Repeat the exercise 10-15 times. (Fig. 10-76)

If you have difficulty bending the knee or standing upright steadily, you can lie on your back and try your best to keep the knee close to the chest. (Fig. 10-77)

(2) Turn with twisted knees: Keep the legs together, bend the body into a semi-squating position, hands on the knees, and turn the knees back and forth and to the left and right gently. First turn from the left, then turn from the right, 10-15 times alternately. The movements should be gentle and slow. (Fig. 10-78)

This method helps strengthen the ligaments of the knee joints. It not only helps improve the bending and extension of the joints, but also relieves pain in the knees. It also has a certain curative effect in treating chronic rheumatic arthritis.

(3) Squat with bent knees: Stand with legs apart at shoulder width, hands on the knees, and squat down slowly. After a slight pause, rise slowly. Keep the buttocks as close as possible to the shanks while squatting. Repeat the movements 5-10 times. (Fig. 10-79)

This method helps strenghten the leg muscles.

If you persevere in doing these exercises they will produce certain curative effect, which may be even better if you also take the proper medicine at the same time. But mind you, do not do them when you have an injury, acute rheumatism, or swollen knee joints. If you have meniscus sprain or softened kneecaps, you should go to a surgeon for advice.

17. Exercises for spasms of the gastrocnemius muscles

Anemia sufferers, people in poor health, those suffering from gastritis, vomiting and loose bowels, and people attacked by sud-

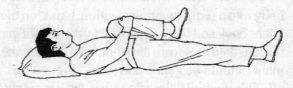

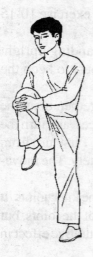

Fig. 10-76

Fig. 10-77

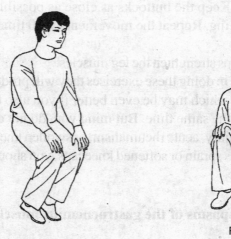

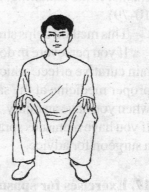

Fig. 10-78

Fig. 10-79

den cold are all subject to muscle spasms. Traditional Chinese medicine believes that deficiency of both *qi* (vital energy) and blood is the internal cause, and attack by wind-cold is the external cause of these spasms. The muscles are less nourished when the vital energy and blood are insufficient, and you have spasms if they are attacked by the wind-cold. Because the four limbs are the parts most easily attacked by wind-cold, the spasms mostly occur in the hands and feet, most often to the lower limbs.

There are many traditional ways of preventing and treating muscle spasms. The easiest and simplest of them is to stretch the limbs. As recorded in the *General Treatise on the Etiology and Symptomology of Diseases*, a famous medical treatise of the Sui Dynasty, one of these ways is to "lie on the back to stretch the legs and hands, heels outward, fingers facing each other, breathing in through the nose seven times. This alleviate rheumatism in the knees, bone ache, and muscle spasm."

It is done this way:

(1) Lie on the back: Stretch the legs and hands, heels apart, toes touching each other. (Fig. 10-80) Stretch the four limbs as energetically as possible. The purpose of keeping the heels apart and touching the toes together is to stretch the muscles of the toes as much as possible.

(2) While stretching the limbs, breathe in through the nose to the maximum, and then breathe out slowly. Do this seven times in a row.

These exercises are intended to stretch the muscles of the limbs. Only if you try your best to stretch them will all the muscles of the limbs be tempered. If you do one to three sessions a day, 5-10 times each session, it will not only help prevent muscle spasms, but will also help alleviate cold knee joints and pain in the shanks. This is very good for people who easily get muscle spasms due to physi-

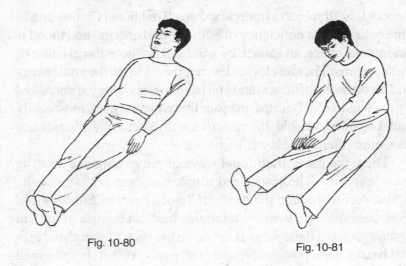

Fig. 10-80   Fig. 10-81

cal weakness and vital energy and blood deficiency.

If you have muscle spasm and cannot bear the pain, you can relieve it by stretching the limbs.

It is done this way:

[1] Straighten the spasaming leg and the toes energetically. Tolerate the pain, do not panic, straighten the limb energetically. If you have difficulty straightening it for a moment, press it down with both hands or with the other leg. If the spasm occurs in the shank, it is good to straighten the shank (Fig. 10-81); if in the toes, it is good to straigthen the toes (Fig. 10-82). The purpose is to stretch and relax the spasaming muscle.

[2] When straightening the limbs, breathe out energetically making a "heh, heh" sound. Be sure to draw a full breath when breathing in, but breathe out forcefully and quickly while making the sounds.

[3] When stretching the limbs, you can also supplement the straightening with some general methods, such as patting the af-

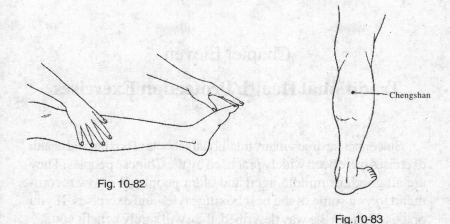

Fig. 10-82

Chengshan

Fig. 10-83

fected part with the hand (pat the shank if the spasm is found in the shank, and pat and massage the muscles of the outer side of the shank if it occurs in the toes), or massage the Chengshan acupoint. (Fig. 10-83)

This method helps alleviate the spasm and also removes muscle contraction. This does not mean you should do the exercises only when there is a spasm. At any time it can help relax the limbs, and is also an effective emergency measure for those who have spasms while swimming.

If the spasm is caused by physical weakness, anemia or low calcium content in the blood, one should go to the doctor for proper treatment, such as toning the blood and increasing the calcium content. If it is caused by excessive vomiting or diarrhea, please consult the doctor in time to replenish the lost blood.

Chapter Eleven

Traditional Health Protection Exercises

Since ancient times, many traditional schools of boxing and health exercises have been widely practised by the Chinese peoples. They are all good for middle-aged and older people. We now recommend to you some of the best boxing styles and exercises. If you practise them in the way described, they will surely benefit you.

1. Taiji Quan

Taiji Quan is a traditional Chinese health exercise and a treasured cultural legacy. It consists of three parts: boxing techniques (hand work, eye techniques, body techniques and footwork), the art of Tuna (abdominal deep breathing which gets rid of the stale and takes in the fresh), and Daoyin exercises (bending forward, bending backward and limb movements).

It is quite true when it is said: "Taiji Quan is the treasure of health preservation for middle-aged and old people," or "Taiji Quan is a good cure for chronic diseases." This is because Taiji Quan movements are soft, stable, round, and slow, and are therefore most suitable for older people and those in poor health.

Taiji Quan helps promote blood circulation, strengthen the functions of the heart and lungs, stimulate digestion, absorption and metabolism in the body, improve the nervous system and the functions of the sense organs, strengthen the muscles, bones and joints, and remove obstructions in the channels and colleterals of the meridian system. Practising Taiji Quan for a long time can help prevent and cure diseases and improve health.

Taiji Quan has a history of hundreds of years and includes many different schools, the best-known among them being Chen-style Taiji Quan, Yang-style Taiji Quan, Wu-style Taiji Quan, and Sun-style Taiji Quan. The most popular style, now widely practised and easy to learn, is the "24 Simplified Forms of Taiji Quan" arranged on the basis of the Yang-style. Since the simplified forms have already been popularized and published by the Foreign Languages Press in English, French, German and Spanish, we are not going to write any more about it in this book, but we hope that our readers will learn and practise it enthusiastically, as it will surely help improve your health.

2. Yijin Jing (muscle-transforming exercise)

The Chinese character "Yi" means transforming, "jin" means muscle, and "Jing" means method. "Yijin" means transforming atrophying and loose muscles into strong and solid muscles.

Yijin Jing is an ancient Chinese health exercise. It was widely practised in the past and is still being practised by many people today. Chinese traditional orthopedists and masseurs usually employ it as their basic professional training exercise.

It can be used not only for day-to-day health care, and physical fitness, but also as an exercise for people recovering from bone fractures.

The movements in this set of exercises are energetic and forceful, implying there is softness in hardness, and stillness in movement, and unity of mind and body, namely, using consciousness to direct muscular power. This is truly a good method of tempering and strengthening the muscles.

This exercise consists of 12 forms:

Exercise 1: Keep the hands in front of the chest

Starting form: Stand with feet apart at shoulder width, hands naturally down, waist and back straight. Looking in front with rapt attention.

[1] Raise both arms slowly to a horizontal level, palms facing down and arms straight.

[2] Turn the palms so they face each other, bend the elbows and move the hands slowly backward into a fist-width from the chest, fingertips pointing at each other and palms facing the chest. (Fig. 11-1)

Points for attention: This is the starting form in which the practitioner is required to adjust the body, keeping it upright and naturally relaxed. The mind should be calm and concentrated, and the breathing natural.

Exercise 2: Stretch the arms horizontally at both sides

Starting form: Continue from [2] in Exercise 1.

[1] Grab the ground with the toes, and at the same time turn the palms over to face up.

[2] Raise the heels slightly, toes on the ground. At the same time, move the hands apart to the sides, palms up. (Fig. 11-2)

Points for attention: Move the hands and feet simultaneously. Concentrate the mind on the palms and toes, and breathe naturally.

Exercise 3: Raise hands upward to hold the sky

Starting form: Continue from [2] in Exercise 2.

[1] Raise the hands upward slowly from both sides in an arc, straighten the arms, palms upward and fingers pointing inward as if holding up the sky. At the same time, raise the heels slightly, toes on the ground, clench the teeth, lick the tongue against the upper palate, breathe finely and concentrate the mind on both hands by looking at the hands through the mind. (Fig. 11-3)

[2] Clench the fists, move the hands slowly and energetically back to horizontal level on both sides, and at the same time put the heels down on the ground.

Points for attention: "Looking through the mind at the hands does not mean using your eyes to look at the hands, but it means using your mind to imagine that you are looking at the hands.

Exercise 4: Pick stars

Starting form: Continue from the previous exercise, stand with legs apart and arms raised horizontally on both sides.

[1] Raise the right hand slowly upward, stretch the arm, palm facing down and fingers together with finger tips pointing inward, and raise the head to look up at the right palm on the upper right. At the same time, put the left hand down and keep the back of the hand against the waist. Hold this for a moment, and breathe 3-5 times. (Fig. 11-4)

[2] Raise the left hand and stretch the arm, palm facing down and fingers together pointing inward, and raise the head to look up at the left palm on the upper left. At the same time, put the right hand down and put the back of the hand against the waist. Hold this for a moment, and breathe 3-5 times.

Repeat this exercise 3-5 times.

Points for attention: Keep the eyes on the raised hand, but concentrate the mind on the waist with the other hand. Breathe in and out through the nose, or breathe in through the nose, and breathe out through the mouth. When breathing in, press the hand on the waist gently, and when breathing out, relax the hand. The breathing should be even, fine, and slow.

Exercise 5: Pull the oxtail backward

Starting form: Continue from [2] in the previous exercise.

[1] Move the right hand back from the waist, turn the wrist over and extend the arm to the right forward, hand at shoulder level and

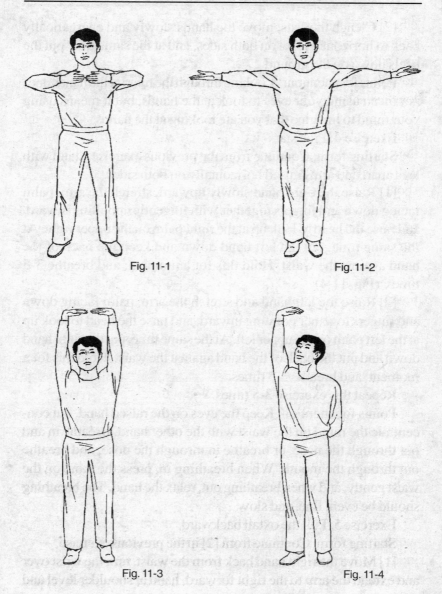

Fig. 11-1

Fig. 11-2

Fig. 11-3

Fig. 11-4

elbow slightly bent, fingers together like a plum blossom to form a hollow fist, fingertips inward. Move the right leg forward, bend it, and straighten the left leg to form a bow stance. Put the left hand down at the same time and extend it to the left backward, fingers together to form a hollow fist, with the fist facing up. (Fig. 11-5)

[2] Breathe in, concentrate the mind on the right hand, move the right hand as if pulling the oxtail backward. Breathe out, concentrate the mind on the left hand, and move the left hand forward as if pulling an ox. Breathe this way several times, with the legs, hands, shoulders and elbows quivering slightly.

[3] Change to the left bow stance, extend the left hand to the left forward. Turn over the wrist and stretch the arm, move the right hand backward to the right and execute the other movements the same way as in [1].

[4] Breathe in and concentrate the mind on the left hand, and breathe out, and concentrate the mind on the right hand. All movements are executed the same way as in [2].

Do the exercise 3-5 times.

Points for attention: While concentrating the mind on the hands, look only through the mind, not the eyes. When breathing, relax the lower abdomen, but move the arms forcefully.

Exercise 6: Push palms and extend arms

Starting form: Continue from [4] in the previous exercise. Move the right foot forward next to the left foot, withdraw both hands to the chest to form the following posture: Stand erect, with the arms bent at elbows by both sides of the chest, fingers apart and palms turned outward.

[1] Turn fingers upward to form an angle of 90 degrees with the wrists, palms outward, and push them slowly forward with the force gradually increasing until the arms are fully extended. At the same time, keep the entire body straight, and open the eyes wide, staring

straight ahead. (Fig. 11-6)

[2] Withdraw the two palms slowly and place them against the ribs on either side of the chest.

Repeat this exercise 3-5 times.

Points for attention: Push the palms forward with light force at first, gradually increasing to strong force. When the palms are entirely pushed out, a large force is exerted as if to push away a mountain. Breathe in when pushing the palms forward, and breathe out when moving them back.

Exercise 7: Draw saber

Starting form: Continue from [2] in the previous exercise. That is, stand erect, raise the arms horizontally forward with the palms facing outward.

[1] Raise the right hand to behind the head and cup the back of the head with the palm, press and pull the left ear with the fingers lightly, open the right armpit, and at the same time, turn the head to the left, and move the left hand backward and place the back of the hand between the shoulder blades. (Fig. 11-7)

[2] Breathe in, and at the same time pull the left ear with the fingers of the right hand, keep the head and the right elbow slightly tense, and concentrate the mind on the elbow. Breathe out and relax. Breathe this way 3-5 times.

[3] Put the right hand down, raise it backhand and place against the back between the shoulder blades. At the same time, withdraw the left hand and raise it to behind the head to cup the back of the head with the palm, press and pull the right ear with the fingers lightly, open the left armpit, and at the same time turn the head to the right.

[4] Breathe out, and at the same time pull the ear with the fingers of the left hand, keep the head and left elbow slightly tense, concentrate the mind on the left elbow. Breathe out and relax. Breathe this

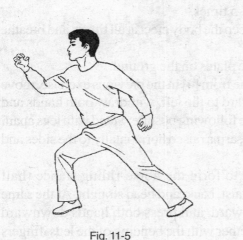

Fig. 11-5

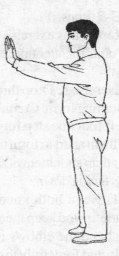

Fig. 11-6

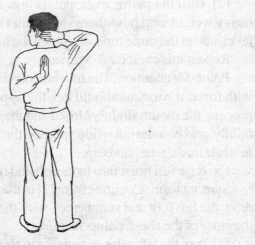

Fig. 11-7

way 3-5 times.

Repeat this exercise 3-5 times.

Points for attention: Keep the body erect at all times, and breathe freely.

Exercise 8: Drop three plates on the ground

Starting form: Continue from [4] in the previous exercise, move the left foot one step forward to the left, withdraw both hands and keep them apart to form the following posture: Stand with legs apart, wider than shoulder width, arms raised horizontally to the sides and palms facing down.

[1] Bend both knees to form the horse-riding stance (half squatting), and keep the waist, back, and head straight. At the same time, bend the elbows inward, and press both hands downward slowly and forcefully together with the bending of the legs, fingers naturally apart with the radial sides inward, and keep them in the air a palm's width right above the knees. (Fig. 11-8)

[2] Turn the palms over, palms upward, as if holding a very heavy weight, and raise them slowly and energetically up to chest level, and at the same time straighten the knees gradually.

Repeat this exercise 3-5 times.

Points for attention: The movements should be slow, steady and with force, the tongue should lick the upper palate throughout the process, the mouth slightly closed and the eyes wide open. Breathe mildly, and breathe out while pressing the hands down and breathe in while raising the hands up.

Exercise 9: Thrust fists to the left and right

Starting form: Continue from [2] in the previous exercise. Withdraw the left foot and stand erect, with the arms bent at elbows by the sides of the chest, palms facing up.

[1] Turn the left palm downward to form a hollow fist and withdraw to the ribs. At the same time, turn the right palm down to form

a hollow fist and thrust it forward to the left. At the same time, turn the head, neck, and waist slightly to the left. (Fig. 11-9)

[2] Withdraw the right fist to by the right ribs. At the same time, thrust the left palm to the right with the rest of the movements being the same as above.

Repeat this exercise 3-5 times.

Points for attention: Withdraw one hand to near the ribs and extend the other hand to the opposite side. Do the two movements at the same time in a coordinated way, with one hand moving forward and one hand moving backward. Breathe in through the nose and breathe out through the mouth. Breathe in while extending the arm and breathe out when the hand is fully extended.

Exercise 10: Fierce tiger springs on prey

Starting form: Continue from [2] in the previous exercise, stand erect, move the hands back with the arms naturally down.

[1] Move the right foot forward to form a right bow step (bend the right knee and straighten the left leg). At the same time, lean the body forward and throw the hands forward and downward, with fingers touching the ground to form the push-up stance, head slightly up, and eyes wide open looking ahead. (Fig. 11-10)

[2] Bend and stretch the elbow joints of both arms gently and slowly. While bending the arms, slink the upper part of the body downward, the chest and head moving slightly forward as if to spring on the prey. While stretching the arms, raise the upper body to its original position, the chest and head moving slightly backward. Repeat this 3-5 times. Then stand up, withdraw the right leg, and return to the starting position.

[3] Move the left foot forward to form a left bow step (bend the left knee and straighten the right leg). At the same time, lean the body forward and throw the hands forward and downward with the essentials of the other movements the same as in [1].

[4] The movements are the same as [2]. Stand up, withdraw the left foot and return to the starting position.

Do this exercise only once.

Points for attention: When throwing the hands forward and downward, relax the waist, keep the spinal column flat and straight, not arched. It is desirable to use the fingertips to touch the ground to support the body. If your finger power is not enough, you can also use your palms. Bend the elbows while breathing. Breathe out while moving the chest forward and breathe in while stretching the elbows and moving the chest back. Breathe in through the nose and breathe out through the mouth.

Exercise 11: Bend the body

Starting position: Continue from [4] in the previous exercise, stand erect with the arms naturally down.

[1] Hold the back of the head with both hands, fingers crossed, palms covering the ears, and stretch the elbows outward with force to shoulder level.

[2] Bend the body forward, head down to knee level, and keep the knees straight. (Fig. 11-11)

[3] Sound the celestial drum: Cover the ears with the palms. With the index fingers on the middle fingers, slip the index fingers down to flick the back of the head (around the Fengchi acupoints) with snapping sounds. Do this 10-12 times.

[4] Raise the body slowly to the standing position, and drop the hands down.

Beginners can do this exercise once or twice, and later do it 3-5 times.

Points for attention: The range of motion while bending the body and keeping the head down differs from person to person. Patients suffering from hypertension or cerebral arteriosclerosis should not do this exercise.

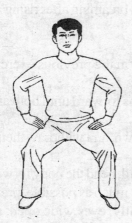

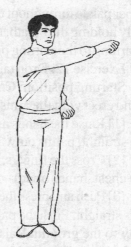

Fig. 11-8

Fig. 11-9

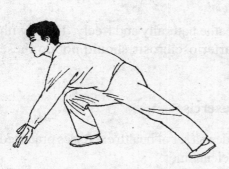

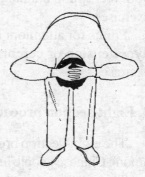

Fig. 11-10

Fig. 11-11

Clench the teeth tightly but lightly with the tongue licking the upper palate throughout the entire exercise. Breathe slightly, practically holding the breath. Return to normal breathing after rising and returning to the starting position.

Exercise 12: Drop tail

Starting position: Continue from [4] in the previous exercise, stand erect with the arms down naturally.

[1] Raise the hands and push the palms forward until both arms are straight, palms outward.

[2] Cross the fingers, palms facing down, and withdraw them to the chest, hands apart.

[3] Push and press the palms downward, bend the body forward, legs straight. Push the palm downward as much as possible, preferably to the ground. Raise the head slightly, eyes wide open, and look ahead (Fig. 11-12)

[4] Stretch the back, rise, and raise the hands at the same time. Extend the arms to both sides seven times. Stamp the ground with both feet (jump and land) seven times to finish the whole set of exercises.

Points for attention: Breathe naturally and freely. Those with hypertension or cerebral arteriosclerosis should not do these exercises.

3. Eight-section brocade exercise

The eight-section brocade is a set of health exercises practised among Chinese people in ancient times.

This set of exercises has been handed down from the Song Dynasty, 800 years ago. It is said to have been created by Yue Fei (1103-1142), a famous Song Dynasty general.

The set consists of eight sections, to be executed as beautifully as brocade, hence the name. There is a pithy formula to help you remember it. The formula is:

Hold up the sky with both hands to regulate the triple energizer,
Draw bows on both sides as if shooting at a vulture.
Regulate the spleen and stomach with one arm raised,
Look backward to relieve five strains and seven harms.
Shake the head and wag the tail to remove heart-fire,
Hold the feet with both hands to strengthen kidneys and waist.
Clench fists with angry eyes to increase physical strength,
Jolt backward seven times behind to cure all diseases.

Since ancient times, people have come to understand the principle that "running water is never stale and a door-hinge never gets worm-eaten." Therefore they improved their physical fitness to prevent illnesses through labor and physical exercises. The eight-section brocade exercise came into being precisely under this guiding thought.

Generally speaking, middle-aged and older people undergo bodily changes through long years of work and daily life with their heads and bodies bent and their backs arched, affecting the functions of their internal organs and nerves and slowly harming their health.

The advantages of the eight-section brocade exercise is that they help increase arm power, regulate the internal organs, and correct the bad posture of drawn shoulders, round back and protruding spinal column. Therefore, it is most suitable for these people.

There are different schools of the eight-section brocade exercise, mainly the civilian school (sitting position) and the military school (standing position). Described below is the military school of the eight-section brocade.

Section 1: Hold up the sky with both hands to regulate the triple energizer

Stand erect, turn the palms outward, raise the arms slowly from both sides, cross the fingers when they are over the head, and turn the palms over to lift them upward, both arms and elbows straight, heels raised as much as possible. At the same time, raise the head, keep eyes at the back of the hands for a moment, and then relax the fingers, put the arms down slowly by the sides of the body and land the heels. Repeat this exercise 3-7 times. (Fig. 11-13)

Section 2: Draw bows on both sides as if shooting at a vulture

Stand erect, move a big step to the left and bend the arms horizontally in front of the chest. Bend the legs to form the horse-riding stance and push the left arm horizontally to the left as if holding a bow, with the index and middle fingers of the left hand raised up, thumb bent and pressed on the ring and little fingers. Bend the right elbow and pull the arm horizontally to the right with the index and middle fingers of the right hand hooked up, as if pulling a string, with the thumb pressed on the ring and little fingers. Look to the left. At the same time, expand the chest and breathe in as if shooting an arrow, and then withdraw both hands and bend the arms in front of the chest and breathe out. Then do the same movements on the right side, in the opposite direction. Shoot the arrows on the two sides alternately, and repeat this many times. (Fig. 11-14)

Section 3: Regulate the spleen and stomach with one arm raised

Stand erect and bend the arms horizontally in front of the chest, fingertips pointing to each other and palms upward. Turn both palms, raise the left arm upward and press the right arm downward at the same time, chest out and waist lowered. Stretch the whole body as much as possible and then restore the arms to the horizontally bent position. Raise the right arm upward and press the left arm downward. Breathe in when raising and pressing the arms, and breathe out when bending the arms. Repeat many times. (Fig. 11-15)

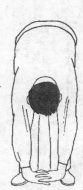

Fig. 11-12

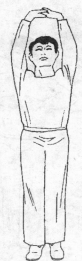

Fig. 11-13

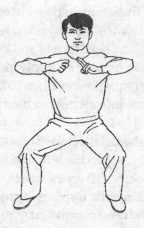

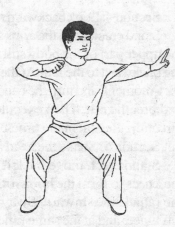

Fig. 11-14

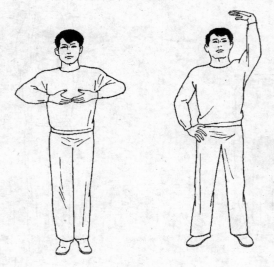

Fig. 11-15

Section 4: Look backward to relieve five strains and seven harms

Stand erect, keep the arms straight down by the two sides. Keep the upper part of the body still with only the head turned and looking backward to the left. At the same time, breathe in deeply, pause for a moment, and turn the head to the original position. Look ahead and breathe out. Then execute the same movements in the right direction. Repeat many times. (Fig. 11-16)

Section 5: Shake the head and wag the tail to remove heart-fire

Stand erect, move the left foot a big step to the left, and bend the knees to form the horse-riding stance, hands on the knees with the radial sides inward. Sway the head and the upper body to the left twice, and at the same time shake the head downward as much as possible and wag the buttocks upward forcefully. First bend and then stretch the left arm, and at the same time stretch first and then

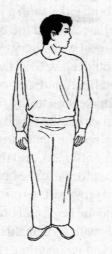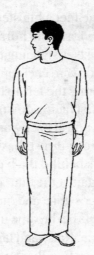

Fig. 11-16

bend the right arm. Then turn the head and the upper body from left to backward and right until the head is bent downward on the right. Then sway the head and the upper part of the body to the right twice, and then turn the head and the upper body from right to forward and left. Finally, stand erect. (Fig. 11-17)

Section 6: Hold the feet with both hands to strengthen kidney and waist

Bend the upper body backward, raise the arms upward and backward, then bend the upper body forward, legs together and knees straight. At the same time, put the hands down forward and hold the feet, bend the upper body further forward, press the hands on the insteps. Then raise the body slightly, and move a bit several times. Then bend the body forward several times. (Fig. 11-18)

Section 7: Clench fists with angry eyes to increase physical strength

Move the feet a big step apart to both sides with a jump, bend the knees to form the horse-riding stance. Bend the elbows and clench the fists, fist facing up. Look ahead with angry eyes. Thrust the left fist forward energetically at shoulder level, fist facing down. Then withdraw the left fist, and thrust the right fist forward at the same time, fist facing down. Repeat this several times. (Fig. 11-19)

Section 8: Jolt backward seven times to cure all diseases

Stand erect, thrust the chest out, place the hands together, and put the arms behind the back, fingers entwined, and the backs of the hands against the buttocks. At the start, raise the heels upward as much as possible, and raise the head upward, toes on the ground. At the same time, breathe in. Then land the heels and breathe out at the same time. Raise and land the heels with a jolt in this way seven or more times. Finally, return to the standing position. (Fig. 11-20)

The number of repititions of these exercises varies from person to person, but you should do enough so that you sweat a bit.

How can the eight-section brocade exercise improve health?

Usually, a gradual change takes place in the circulatory system of middle-aged and older people as their age. For example, the walls of the blood vessels become thickened, their elasticity is weakened, and circulation in the blood capillaries becomes slow. The eight-section brocade exercise helps improve blood circulation. For example, the "triple energizer" in Section 1 is a term for the three different parts of the human body in traditional Chinese medicine. The upper energizer is the thoracic cavity, the middle energizer is the abdominal cavity and the lower energizer is the pelvic cavity. In fact, these stretching movements of the limbs and trunk involves the redistribution of the blood flow in the thoracic cavity and the abdominal cavity and strengthens the contraction of the muscles, thus improving the blood circulation and regulating the in-

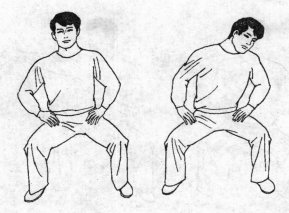

Fig. 11-17

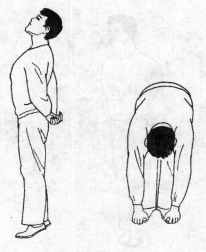

Fig. 11-18

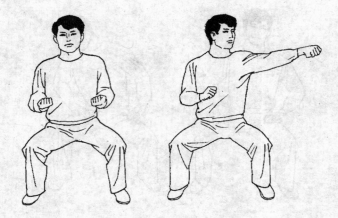

Fig. 11-19

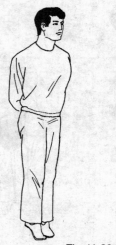

Fig. 11-20

ternal organs.

Older people are subject to senile pulmonary emphysema as a result of the atrophy of the mucous membrane and tissues of the nose. Moreover, the atrophy of the respiratory muscles restricts activity in the thoracic cavity, resulting in the reduction of the vital capacity. This is why older folks easily get palpitations and asthma. The exercise in section 2 helps to expand the lungs, deepen breathing, improve the vital capacity, and increase the content of oxygen in the blood so that the whole body gets a sufficient supply of oxygen. It also helps dissipate fatigue, refresh the mind, and increase vigor. Moreover, it also delays the atrophy and decline of the function of the lungs.

The upward raising of one hand and the downward pressing of the other in section 3, and the energetic pulling in opposite directions help strengthen the peristalsis and secretion of the stomach and intestines, stimulate the appetite, and maintain normal functioning of the digestive system.

The five strains referred to in section 4 are the strains of the heart, liver, spleen, lung and kidney. The seven harms refers to harm done to the seven emotions, and the seven diseases caused by kidney insufficiency. By turning the head left and right repeatedly and looking backward as much as possible, this part of the exercise helps invigorate blood circulation in the head and strengthens the muscles of the neck and cervical vertebra movement. Practice has shown that older people who practise the "eight-section brocade" everyday can maintain a stable blood pressure and alleviate vascular sclerosis.

Section 6 involves bending both forward and backward to help extend the lumbar muscles and strengthen the lumbar tissue. It can not only prevent and treat common lumbar muscle strain, but also strengthen the functions of the entire body.

271

Every movement in the "eight-section brocade" has its purpose.

4. Five animal-mimic exercises

The five animal-mimic exercises were originated by Hua Tuo, a famous physician of the Eastern Han Dynasty (25-220). It was 1,000 years earlier than the medical exercises invented in Sweden.

The five animal-mimic exercises were created on the basis of imitating the movements of five animals—the fierceness of the tiger in springing on prey, the stretching of the neck of the deer, the stable and steady walking of the bear, the nimble leap of the monkey, and the flying of the bird.

Through the long years of the development, these exercises have become divided into many different schools.

The following is a description of the best set of exercises, chosen for our readers, simple and easy to learn. Our readers may practise them all or in part.

(1) Bear form

[1] Starting position: Stand naturally with feet parallel and apart at shoulder width, and arms naturally down. (Fig. 11-21) After breathing deeply 3-5 times, sway the waist and arms naturally.

[2] Bend the right knee, sway the right shoulder downward and drop the arm. Stretch the left shoulder slightly backward and outward, and raise the left arm up slightly. (Fig. 11-22)

[3] Bend the left knee, sway the left shoulder forward and downward and drop the arm. Stretch the right shoulder backward slightly and out, and raise the right arm slightly higher. (Fig. 11-23)

Sway the shoulders in this way repeatedly, as many times as you like. This helps strengthen the spleen and stomach, promote digestion and invigorate the joints. The essentials are: Sway the shoulders and twist the waist naturally, keep the joints as loose as cotton, grab the ground flexibly and steadily, and regulate the vital energy and keep it in the Dantian region.

(2) Tiger form

[1] Starting position: Keep the arms naturally down, the neck naturally upright, the face natural, the eyes looking ahead, the mouth closed, and the tongue lightly licking the upper palate. Do not thrust the chest out nor arch the back. Put the heels together to form an angle of 90 degrees and stand erect. Relax the entire body, and stand in this way for a while. (Fig. 11-24)

[2] Left form: a. Bend the legs slowly downward into a half squatting position, and shift the body weight to the right leg. Place the left foot by the right ankle joint, left heel slightly off the ground and ball touching the ground. At the same time, clench the fists and raise them on both sides, fist facing up. Look ahead and to the left. (Fig. 11-25)

b. Move the left foot one step obliquely forward to the left, with the right foot following half a step forward, heel to heel, 30 cm apart. Keep the body weight on the right leg and form a left empty step. At the same time, extend the fists upward along the chest, fists facing inward, and turn them inward and change into palms when at mouth level. Then press the palms forward to chest level, palms facing forward with the radial sides opposite each other. Look at the index finger of the left hand. (Fig. 11-26)

[3] Right form: a. Skip the left foot half a step forward, and move the right foot immediately behind to the ankle joint of the left foot, legs close to each other, the right heel slightly off and the right ball touching the ground. Bend the legs to a half squatting position to form a left single leg stance. At the same time, change the palms into fists and draw them back to the sides of the waist, fists facing up. Look ahead and to the right. (Fig. 11-27)

b. Move the right foot obliquely forward to the right, with the

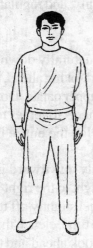

Fig. 11-21

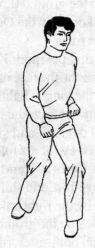

Fig. 11-22

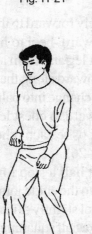

Fig. 11-23

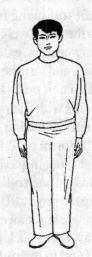

Fig. 11-24

left foot moving immediately half a step forward, heels opposite each other and about 30 cm apart. Keep the body weight on the left leg to form the right empty step. At the same time, extend the fists along the chest upward, fists facing inward, then turn them over and change into palms when extended to mouth level and press them forward to chest level, palms facing forward, the radial sides facing each other. Look at the index finger of the right hand. (Fig. 11-28)

[4] Left form: a. Skip the right foot half a step forward, and move the left foot immediately behind to the ankle joint of the right foot, heel slightly off and the ball slightly touching the ground. Bend the legs to a half squatting position to form a right single stance. At the same time, change the palms into fists and draw them back to both sides, fists facing up. Look ahead and to the left. (Fig. 11-25)

b. All movements are the same as in b. of [2] Left Form described above. (Fig. 11-26)

Do the tiger exercise this way, on both sides. The number of times is not limited. The movements should be coordinated and quick, calm, and fierce.

(3) Monkey form

[1] The starting position is the same as that in the tiger form.

[2] Bend the legs slowly downward, move the left foot lightly and nimbly forward. At the same time, when the left hand is raised along the chest up to mouth level, stretch it forward as if grabbing something, and change the hand into a claw when nearly to the final point. Bend the wrist down naturally. (Fig. 11-29)

[3] Move the right foot lightly and nimbly forward, with the left foot following slightly, heel off and ball touching the ground lightly. At the same time, when the right hand is raised along the chest up to mouth level, stretch it forward as if grabbing something, and change the hand into a claw when nearly to the final point. At the same time, withdraw the right hand to under the right ribs. (Fig. 11-30)

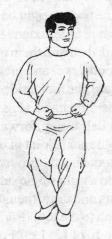

Fig. 11-25

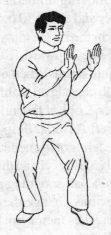

Fig. 11-26

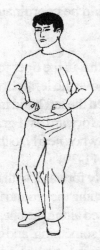

Fig. 11-27

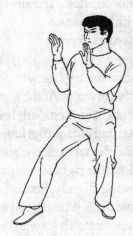

Fig. 11-28

[4] Move the left foot slightly backward and stand firm, move the body to sit back, move the right foot slightly backward immediately, toes touching the ground. At the same time, when the left hand is raised along the chest to mouth level, stretch it forward as if grabbing something, and change the hand into a claw when nearly at the final point. Bend the wrist downward immediately and at the same time withdraw the right hand to under the right ribs. (Fig. 11-31)

[5] Move the right foot lightly and nimbly forward, and at the same time, when the right hand is raised along the chest to mouth level, stretch it forward as if grabbing something, and change the hand into a claw when nearly at the final point. Bend the wrist down naturally. (Fig. 11-32)

[6] Move the left foot lightly and nimbly forward, with the right foot following slightly, heel off and toes touching the ground slightly. At the same time, when the left hand is raised along the chest to mouth level, stretch it forward as if grabbing something, and change the hand into a claw when nearly to the final point. Bend the wrists down naturally. At the same time, withdraw the right hand to under the right ribs. (Fig. 11-33)

[7] Move the right foot slightly backward and stand firm. Move the body to sit back, move the left foot also lightly backward, toes touching the ground. At the same time, when the right hand is raised along the chest to mouth level, stretch it forward as if grabbing something, and change the hand into a claw when nearly to the final point. Bend the wrist down naturally. At the same time, withdraw the left hand to under the left ribs. (Fig. 11-31, opposite to the left)

(4) Deer form

[1] Bend the right leg, sit the upper body back, left leg extended forward, knee slightly bent, left foot touching the ground slightly to form the left empty step.

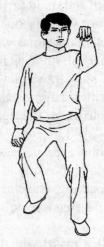

Fig. 11-29

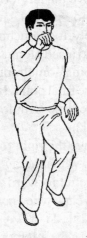

Fig. 11-30

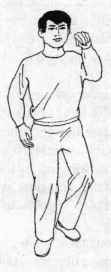

Fig. 11-31

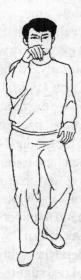

Fig. 11-32

[2] Extend the left hand, elbow slightly bent. Place the right hand by the inner side of the left elbow, palms opposite to each other.

[3] Rotate both arms counterclockwise simultaneously, the left hand moving in a larger circle than the right hand. The essential point is that the circle is not drawn around the shoulder joints, but around the waist and hips. The arms draw big circles while the coccyx draws small circles. This is what is known as "deer moves the coccyx." It is mainly intended to invigorate the waist and hips in order to strengthen the kidneys, promote the blood circulation in the pelvic cavity, and increase leg power. (Fig. 11-34)

[4] After circling several times like this, move the right leg forward, sit the upper body on the left leg, extend the right hand forward with the left hand protecting the right elbow, and circling around clockwise several times. Do this exercise on the left and right alternately.

(5) Bird form

[1] Starting position: Stand with feet together, arms down naturally, and look ahead. Stand calmly for a while.

[2] Move the left foot one step forward, with the right foot following half a step immediately and toes touching the ground slightly. At the same time, raise both arms in front of the body to both sides, and breathe in deeply. (Fig. 11-35)

[3] Move the right foot forward to the side of the left foot, drop the arms on both sides, cross the hands under the knees and breathe out deeply at the same time. (Fig. 11-36)

[4] Move the right foot one step forward, with the left foot following half a step forward and toes touching the ground slightly. At the same time, raise both arms in front of the body to both sides, and breathe in deeply. (Fig. 11-37)

(5) Move the left foot forward to the side of the right foot, drop the arms on both sides, cross the hands under the knees and breathe out deeply at the same time. (Fig. 11-36)

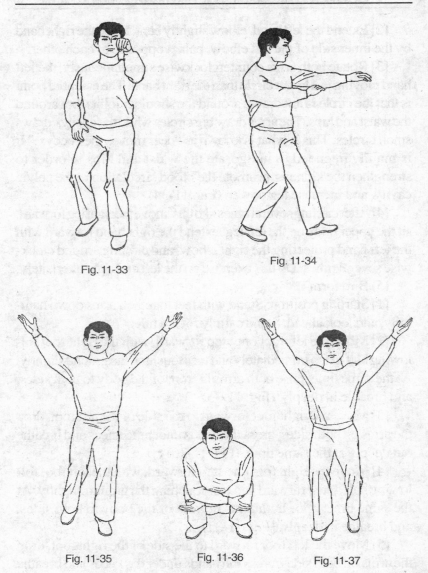

Fig. 11-33

Fig. 11-34

Fig. 11-35

Fig. 11-36

Fig. 11-37

This exercise helps improve the function of the heart and lungs and strengthens the kidneys and waist. If you persist in doing it everyday, it also helps cure lumbar pains.

The "*gong*" in *qigong* refers to the exercises being practised or the skill of the practitioner.

To practise *qigong* is to train the body through the methods of *qigong*, and by all methods of conscious control, to become filled with sufficient energy and ensure its smooth flow for invigorating the functions of metabolism and immunity, while tapping the potentials for life maintenance.

This chapter describes some simple, easy-to-learn, and effective practical *qigong* exercises. Before getting down to business, we would like to give you an understanding of some basic questions involved:

(1) How to learn to practise *qigong*

First of all, believe that *qigong* is a science. A common saying goes: "If you are sincere, it is effective." The attitude of the Chinese is: "If you believe in it, it is effective. If you do not believe in it, it is not effective." This is because *qigong* produces its effect only when the cerebrum falls into quiescence through mental concentration. If you have any doubt, it is difficult to get into the best state of mind.

Second, have confidence and determination. Since *qigong* is the crystallization of the activities of human life, everybody can learn to practise it. However, if you are not very determined or if you practise only now and then, or practise *qigong* just to follow the fashion or to hunt for novelty, it is absolutely impossible to learn to do it well, and you will get nothing from it.

Third, practise with perseverance. You must make unremitting efforts. If you practise in an orderly, step by step way, you will surely benefit. No matter what difficulty you might encounter, you should practise with perseverance and patience. Once you have made the efforts, you will reap the results. You should take the time to preserve your good health and practise regularly everyday.

Fourth, do not practise blindly, but rather earnestly and in the way you are taught, because the wrong way will only bring you trouble.

(2) Essentials for practising *qigong*

There are many kinds of *qigong* exercises and there are also many ways to practise *qigong*. There are three types of *Qigong*: dynamic *qigong*, static *qigong*, and dynamic-static *qigong*. However, no matter which *qigong* you practise, you must adjust your breathing, fall into quiescence and focus your attention.

There are many essential principals for practising *qigong*, but the most fundamental of these are: adjusting posture, adjusting breathing and adjustment of mental activities (psychological state).

[1] Adjusting posture: Usually, people practise *qigong* in sitting, lying, standing or walking postures. Whichever posture you choose, you should relax, fall into quiescence, and be natural to invigorate the smooth flow of the *qi* (vital energy) and blood. Only in this way can you relax and enable the cerebral cortex to fall into a protective state of inhibition quickly. Usually, when practising sitting *qigong* or lying *qigong*, the consumption of oxygen in the body is reduced and the body is in a physiological state of low metabolism. In order to adjust your posture, you must not be impatient or too relaxed, but keep the body erect with the head and neck upright.

[2] Adjusting breathing: After assuming a posture, you should immediately adjust your breathing. Great attention should be paid to breathing when practising *qigong*. The general requirements are: breathe naturally, evenly, slowly, deeply, calmly, finely and silently. Most people use the abdominal breathing method, including both the orthodromic and counter-moving methods. In the former, the abdomen is dilated while breathing in, and contracted while breathing out. In the latter, the abdomen is contracted while breathing in, and dilated while breathing out. Abdominal breathing helps promote the peristalsis of the stomach and intestines and is therefore

good for improving absorption and digestion and increasing the appetite. It is effective for massaging the internal organs and adjusting their functions.

[3] Adjusting mental activities: After adjusting posture and breathing, it is necessary to adjust mental activities. It is very important to relax the mind and stabilize the emotions, and to keep calm, dispel distracting thoughts, and fall quickly into quiescence. The way to induce the mind to fall into quiescence is to concentrate the mind on the lower abdomen. That is, concentrate the mind on the Dantian accupoint or elixir field (Dantian is located 5 cm below the navel) where *qi* is stored. When the mind is concentrated, it seems to use Dantian to listen to your breathing. That is, using one thought to dispel all distracting thoughts. By this time, the lower abdomen is filled with blood and becomes heated and the central nerves can be inhibited. As you breathe, the internal organs are in a state of movement. In the words of modern medicine, the cerebral cortex enters into a state of inhibition so that the cerebrum is at rest. This helps restore the cells of the cerebral cortex which has been thrown into disorder by over-excitation and pathological excitors. This provides the conditions for resisting diseases and restoring health.

(3) Points for attention

Attention should be paid to the following points for all methods of *qigong*:

[1] Dispel all distracting thoughts and keep calm. You should not practise *qigong* when you are upset, in a bad mood, or very nervous.

[2] Practise *qigong* in a quiet place early in the morning or in the evening when it is quiet.

[3] Watch what you eat and improve your nutrition. Do not eat too much or too little before you practise *qigong*. Under normal conditions, do not practise *qigong* when you are full or hungry, and

do not eat raw, cold, sour, hot or very pungent food.

[4] Lead a regular life, adjust your sleep and control your sexual activity properly.

[5] Avoid catching cold, uproars, cries and other noises. Do not talk with others, and keep quiet.

[6] Pay attention to the closing form of the *qigong* exercises. You must close the form before you end the exercises, and you must have consciousness before closing the form. You just say silently three times: "I am now closing the form." You must keep calm and open your eyes slowly at this time. Do not do strenuous exercises or stand in the wind when you are closing the exercises.

(4) Effect

After practising *qigong* for a while, your body will produce some special effects. One type is a normal effect, and the other an abnormal effect.

Signs of normal effects are:

[1] An ease of mind, slight sweating, and sense of numbness and distention in the limbs.

[2] Slightly itching skin as if an insect is creeping.

[3] A slight stirring in the muscles and cracking in the joints.

[4] Sober-mindedness, full vigor, and sound sleep.

[5] Quicker peristalsis of the intestines and stomach, with a stronger appetite and good digestion.

Of course, not everyone will have all these effects. They may have one, two or three, and only those who practise *qigong* perfectly will realize all of these effects.

Attention should be paid to any of the following adverse effects should they occur after doing *qigong* for a while:

[1] Feeling muddle-headed, listless, dizzy or insomnia. This may be caused by excessive tension and mental strain.

[2] Palpitations with an oppressed feeling in the chest. This may

be caused by improper posture and breathing.

[3] Distention of the abdomen with *qi* surging upward from the lower abdomen. This is usually caused by improper breathing and mental strain.

[4] Itching throat and dry mouth. This is caused by improper breathing, a tightly closed mouth or breathing with the mouth open.

If any of these conditions appear while practising *qigong*, you should find the cause as early as possible and take measures to avoid harmful consequences.

2. The *qigong* exercises you can do

We just recommend some simple and effective *qigong* exercises for your choice.

(1) Inner health cultivation exercise

The inner health cultivation exercise is a *qigong* exercise for strengthening the body and adjusting the internal organs. It is good for the digestive and respiratory systems and is characterized by stillness of the cerebrum and movement of the internal organs.

[1] Postures: Lying on the side, lying supine, sitting, and zhuang-style.

a. Lying on the side: Lie on the side on the bed, bend the head forward slightly with the height of the head adjusted by the pillow. Keep the neck in a slightly higher upright position. Bend the spinal column slightly forward with the chest drawn in and the back straightened. If you lie on the right side, keep the right arm bent naturally, fingers stretched, palm facing up placed on the pillow in front. Keep the left arm naturally straight, fingers loosely apart and palm downward placed on the hip on the same side. Keep the right leg naturally straight and the left leg bent at knee to an angle of 120 degrees and the left knee lightly on the right knee. If lying on the left side, the positions of the body parts are reversed. Close the eyes lightly or open them slightly. Open and close the mouth as required by the breathing methods (see below). (Fig. 12-1)

b. Lying-supine: Lie supine on the bed, body straight and arms stretched naturally, fingers loosely apart, palms downward or inward by both sides. Keep the legs naturally straight, heels together and tiptoes naturally apart. The movements of the mouth and eyes are the same as when lying on the side. (Fig. 12-2)

c. Sitting: Sit up straight in a chair, bend the head slightly forward, body upright, chest drawn in, back straight, shoulders relaxed, elbows down, fingers relaxed, palms downward on the knees, feet parallel to each other and apart to shoulder width, shanks perpendicular to the ground and knees bent to an angle of 90 degrees. If the chair is too high or too low, put something under your buttocks or feet to make adjustments. The movements of the mouth and eyes are the same as when lying on the side. (Fig. 12-3)

4. Zhuang-style: The movements are the same as in the lying-supine position, but the pillow should be 25 cm higher. Put some clothes under your shoulders to form a slope so that the back is not suspended. Keep the feet together, and the palms inward and tight against the sides of the thighs. All other movements are the same as in the lying-supine position. (Fig. 12-4)

In practising the inner health cultivation exercise, beginners usually start with the lying postures. Which lying posture should be used depends on the individual. Generally speaking, a person with lower tension, strong peristalsis and slow discharge should choose the right side lying posture, especially after meals. Those with ptosis of the gastric mucous membrane should not use the right side lying posture because it will aggravate this condition. The lying and sitting postures can be used together or singly. The zhuang-style is also a lying posture, but is usually used after practising *qigong* for some time to

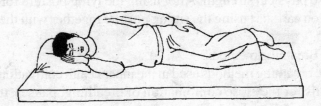

Fig. 12-1

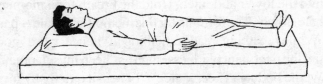

Fig. 12-2

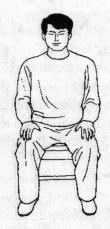

Fig. 12-3

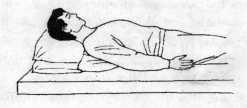

Fig. 12-4

increase physical strength. After using the lying posture for some days, you can start using the sitting posture together with the lying posture.

[2] Breathing methods:

The breathing methods used in the inner health cultivation exercise calls for the close combination of breathing, pauses, tongue movement, and reading in silence. There are three common methods:

a. Close the mouth lightly and breathe through the nose. Inhale first and at the same time use the mind to guide the flow of the breath into the lower abdomen. Hold the breath for a moment and then exhale slowly. The formula for this method is: Inhale—pause—exhale. While breathing, read something in silence, words good for health and the treatment of illness, such as "keep myself quiet," "relax the whole body and keep quiet," "better sit quietly by myself," "keep the internal organs in motion and the cerebrum in quiescence," "cultivate genuine energy to cure all illnesses," "practise *qigong* in earnest to improve health," and "perseverance keeps me in good health."

While reading in silence, combine it closely with breathing and tongue movement. For example, when you read "zi ji jing"(keep myself quiet), read "zi" while inhaling, "ji" while pausing, and "jing" while exhaling. As for tongue movement, this means the rise and fall of the tongue. When breathing in, stick the tongue against the upper palate. Keep the tongue stuck there during the pause, and drop it when exhaling. Practise this way until the cerebrum falls into quiescence, and then stop reading.

b. Breathe through the nose or through both the nose and the mouth. First breathe in without pause, and then breathe out slowly. Pause after exhaling. The formula for this method is: Inhale-exhale-pause. Read the same words in silence as in the first method, but read the first character "zi" while inhaling, "ji" while exhaling, and the other characters while pausing. Stick the tongue against the upper palate when breathing in, drop it when exhaling. Do not move the tongue when pausing.

c. Breathe through the nose. First breathe in a bit, pause immediately, and then breathe in again, stick the tongue against the upper palate and at the same time read the first character "zi" in silence. Stick the tongue against the upper palate and read the second character in silence while pausing. Then breathe in strongly and use the mind to guide the flow of breath into the lower abdomen, and at the same time read the third character in silence. Do not pause after breathing in, but breathe out slowly and drop the tongue. Repeat. The formula for this method is: Inhale-pause- inhale-exhale. In using this method, only read words with three characters.

Why read in silence when practising the inner health cultivation exercise? Because reading in silence helps to keep your mind concentrated and dispels distracting thoughts. At the same time, the suggestion and guidance by words produce a physiological effect corresponding to the words. Therefore, the choice of characters or words should differ from person to person, and from illness to illness. For example, a person with chronic tension should choose "wo song jing" (keep myself relaxed and calm) while a person with a poor spleen may choose to read "nei zang dong, da nao jing" (keep the internal organs in motion and the cerebrum in quiessence). The number of characters read in silence should be small at the beginning and increased gradually as your breathing becomes fine and mild. Silent reading is only supplementary to the breathing exercise, it is not used to control breathing speed or duration.

[3] Mind concentration methods:

Mind concentration refers to concentrating the mind on a certain thing or a certain image while practising *qigong*. Mind concentration helps dispel distracting thoughts, and is an important element of *qigong*. It must be practised well.

There are three methods of mind concentration in the inner health cultivation exercise:

a. Concentrate the mind on Dantian: Dantian is a common term used in *qigong* exercises. It is 5 cm below the navel and is where the Qihai acupoint is located. It was believed in ancient times that Dantian was "the source of *qi* and the place where *qi* is stored." When the mind is concentrated on Dantian, the primordial energy is strong and all diseases are resisted. This means that full attention is focused on the lower abdomen. Just imagine a circular area or a spheroid with the Qihai acupoint as its center. As time goes by, you will feel warmth in the lower abdomen whenever you practise *qigong*.

b. Concentrate the mind on the Danzhong acupoint: Danzhong is located in the middle of the chest between the breasts. While the mind is concentrated there, just imagine a circular area with the Shanzhong acupoint as its center between the breasts.

c. Concentrate the mind on the toes: Close the eyes gently with a ray of light and the mind following the line of vision. Focus attention on the big toe and imagine the image of the toe.

Generally, concentrating the mind on Dantian is safer, and without side effects to the head, chest or abdomen. The rhythmic rise and fall of the abdominal wall arising from the exercise, coupled with breathing, helps concentrate the mind and dispel distracting thoughts. If some women experience more menstrual bleeding or a longer menstrual period, they should use the method of concentrating the mind on the Danzhong acupoint. People with distracting thoughts have difficulty concentrating their mind on Dantian with eyes closed, and instead can concentrate their mind on the toes.

No matter which method is used, it should be done naturally.

(2) Health promotion exercise

The health promotion exercise has been developed on the basis of the inner health cultivation exercise by absorbing the best of the schools of Buddhism, Taoism, Confucianism and secular methods. This has an ideal effect in improving physical conditions, maintaining health, and prolonging life. A description of the exercise follows:

[1] Posture: Sitting posture (sitting with legs naturally bent, one leg crossed or both legs crossed), standing posture and free posture.

a. Sitting with legs naturally bent: Keep the shanks crossed, soles backward and out, buttocks on the mattress, and thighs on the shanks. Keep the head, neck and upper body upright, and the buttocks slightly back so that the chest is slightly drawn in. Relax the cervical muscles, lean the head slightly forward, close the eyes lightly, and drop the arms naturally. Keep hands together or put one hand on the palm of the other, and put them on the thighs in front of the abdomen. (Fig. 12-5)

b. Sitting with one leg crossed: Sit with the legs crossed, left shank on top of the right shank, with the left instep tightly on the right thigh and the sole upward. Or the right shank on top of the left shank, with the right instep tightly on the left thigh and the sole upward. All other movements are the same as in a. (Fig. 12-6)

c. Sitting with both legs crossed: Keep the right shank on top of the left shank and put the left shank on top of the right shank so that the two shanks cross each other, both soles upward and placed on the thighs. All other movements are the same as above. (Fig. 12-7)

The three sitting postures may easily cause numbness in the legs, but they help you fall into quiescence. If you have difficulty with this while doing the exercise, just stretch the legs or use the hands to massage them, and the legs will recover. Then change to another posture and continue.

d. Standing posture: Stand with feet apart at shoulder width, bend the knees slightly, draw the chest in, keep the spinal column upright, lean the head slightly forward, close the eyes slightly, relax the shoulders, and drop the elbows and bend the forearms slightly. Keep both thumbs apart from the other fingers as if holding something in front of the lower abdomen. (Fig. 12-8) Or raise the forearms upward and put the hands in front of the chest as if holding a ball. (Fig. 12-9)

Practise the standing posture either indoors or outdoors, but it is best to choose a quiet place with fresh air.

e. Free posture: You are not required to use any fixed posture. It just depends on the situation when you practise *qigong*.

[2] Breathing methods: Static breathing, deep breathing, beat-counting breathing, and converse breathing.

a. Static breathing: This is also called natural breathing. Breathe naturally when practising *qigong*. You are not required to change your normal breathing nor use consciousness to guide your breathing. However, it is still different from regular breathing. Breathe when the body is relaxed, distracting thoughts are dispelled, and the mind is calm and quiet. This has the effect of adjusting breathing and mental activities. This method is most suitable for older and physically weak people, and people suffering from lung diseases.

b. Deep breathing: This is also called mixed deep and long breathing. Breathe as deeply and as long as possible to expand your vital capacity. When breathing in, both the chest and abdomen should bulge, the breathing is quiet, fine, even, gentle and slow. When the cerebrum falls into quiescence, the breathing becomes continuous and unbroken, as though stopping, but still existing. This method is best suited for people suffering from neurosis, constipation or absent-mindedness.

c. Beat-counting breathing: Do not count the number of times when breathing in, but count the number of times when breathing out. When you count to 10, start counting again from the beginning. This method is good for stilling the mind. Stop counting after the

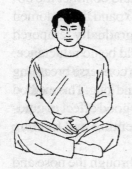
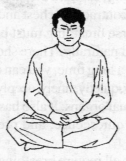
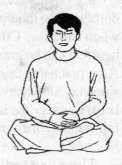

Fig. 12-5   Fig. 12-6   Fig. 12-7

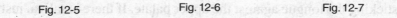

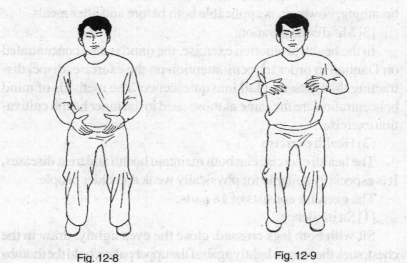
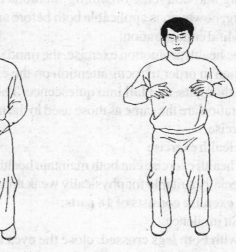

Fig. 12-8   Fig. 12-9

cerebrum becomes quiet.

d. Converse breathing: Expand the chest and contract the abdomen when inhaling; contract the chest and expand the abdomen when exhaling. Converse breathing must be gradually tempered before it can be grasped naturally. There should be no reluctance. After practising this for a long time, you can do converse breathing smoothly, slowly, evenly, quietly, finely, deeply and long. This method helps massage the internal organs. It also has a good effect in guiding the cerebrum into quiescence, and preventing and treating illnesses.

These four methods all require breathing through the nose and sticking the tongue against the upper palate. If there is saliva, just swallow it down slowly. If there is anything wrong with your nose, just open your mouth a bit to help breathing. Do not use the deep breathing and converse breathing methods after meals. Static breathing, however, is applicable both before and after meals.

[3] Mind concentration:

In the health promotion exercise, the mind is also concentrated on Dantian in order to focus attention on the exercise, dispel distracting thoughts, and fall into quiescence. The methods of mind concentration are the same as those used in the inner health cultivation exercise.

(3) Health exercise

The health exercise can both maintain health and treat diseases. It is especially suitable for physically weak and older people.

The exercise consists of 18 parts:

[1] Sit in silence:

Sit with both legs crossed, close the eyes lightly, draw in the chest, stick the tongue lightly against the upper palate, hold the thumbs with your fingers and put them on the thighs. (Fig. 12-10)

Concentrate the mind on Dantian and breathe through the nose

50 times. Beginners may use the natural breathing method, but gradually deepen it as time goes on, or use the deep breathing or abdominal breathing method.

Sitting in silence helps to calm the mood, dispel distracting thoughts, relax the muscles and tranquilize breathing, thus preparing for practising the following exercises. This exercise requires deep breathing 50 times to improve the lungs absorption of oxygen and carbon discharge. This helps improve blood circulation throughout the body.

[2] Ear exercise (sound the celestial drum):

Massage the helices respectively with both hands 18 times (Fig. 12-11), cover the external auditory meatuses with the thenar of the hands, with the fingers on the back of the head (Fig. 12-12), press the middle fingers with the index fingers, and slip them down to flick the back of the head 24 times with the sounds of rub-a-dab (sound the celestial drum). (Fig. 12-13)

Massaging the helices helps stimulate the auditory nerves and increase its excitation, improves hearing ability and prevents and treats tinnitus and deafness. The ear exercise helps give mild and soft stimulation to the cerebrum and adjusts the function of the central nerve. At the same time, it also helps stimulate the circulatory center and improves the function of the heart and lungs and helps relieve headaches and dizziness.

[3] Click the teeth:

Concentrate the mind and click the upper and lower teeth together lightly 36 times.

This helps stimulate the teeth, improves the blood circulation around the teeth, keeps them firm and prevents dental disease.

[4] Tongue exercise:

Move the tongue up and down inside the mouth and outside the teeth and from left to right 18 times, and then from right to left 18

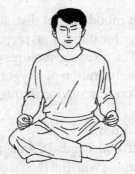

Fig. 12-10

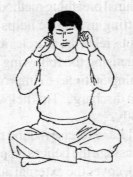

Fig. 12-11

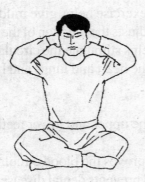

Fig. 12-12

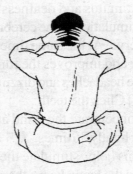

Fig. 12-13

times. Saliva comes out by this time, so rinse the mouth with the saliva before swallowing it.

[5] Rinse the mouth with saliva:

Close the mouth, and rinse the mouth 36 times with the saliva produced during the tongue exercise, and then swallow it in three separate actions with gurgling sounds. Use the mind to guide the saliva slowly down through to Dantian.

The tongue exercise and mouth rinsing with saliva helps stimulate the secretion of the digestive glands so that the intestinal fluid secreted increases to improve the digestive function, increase the appetite and promote the absorption of nutriments.

[6] Rub the nose:

First warm the backs of the thumbs by rubbing (Fig. 12-14), pinch the nose with the backs of the thumbs, and rub the two sides of the nose lightly (with the Yingxiang acupoints as the centers) 18 times on each side. (Fig. 12-15)

This exercise helps increase the resistance of the upper respiratory tract, and has the effect of preventing you from catching cold. It also helps treat chronic nose diseases and allergic rhinitis and has an instant effect in relieving a stuffy nose.

[7] Eye exercise:

Close the eyes lightly, bend the thumbs slightly, rub the eyelids lightly with the finger joints 18 times on each side (Fig. 12-16), and then rub the eyebrows lightly with the backs of the thumbs 18 times on each side. (Fig. 12-17) Then, close the eyes lightly again and let the eyeballs turn to left and right inside the eye sockets 18 times each.

This exercise helps promote the movements of the eyeballs and eye muscles, accelerate the blood circulation in the eyes, prevent eye diseases, and improve eyesight.

[8] Rub the face:

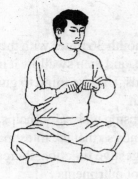

Fig. 12-14

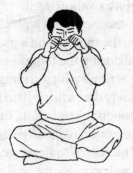

Fig. 12-15

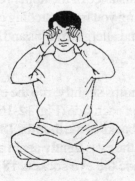

Fig. 12-16

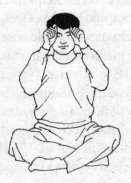

Fig. 12-17

Warm both palms by rubbing them together, then rub the face with both palms from the forehead downward along both sides of the nose (Fig. 12-18) to the lower chin, and then from the lower chin upward to the forehead. (Fig. 12-19) Rub the face up and down this way 36 times.

[9] Neck Exercise:

Cross the fingers of both hands and hold the back of the neck, look up (Fig. 12-20), and then pull the hands forward while bending, massage the neck backward, do this 3-9 times. (Fig. 12-21)

This exercise helps to relieve shoulder pain and dizziness, and promote blood circulation.

[10] Rub the shoulders:

First rub the left shoulder with the right palm 18 times (Fig. 12-22), and then rub the right shoulder with the left palm 18 times. (Fig. 12-23)

This exercise helps promote blood circulation in the shoulder, and cure and prevent inflammation of the shoulder joints and areas around the shoulder joints.

[11] Jiaji exercise:

Clench the fists lightly, bend the arms to an angle of 90 degrees at the elbows, and swing the arms back and forth alternately 18 times on each side. (Figs. 12-24, 12- 25)

[12] Rub the waist (rub the internal kidneys):

First rub warm the hands and then rub the two sides of the waist with the warm hands 18 times on each side. (Fig. 12-26)

This exercise helps promote blood circulation in the waist, remove fatigue from the lumbar muscles, and prevent and cure lumbago, dysmenorrhea and amenorrhea.

[13] Rub the coccyx:

Rub the two sides of the coccyx with the index and middle fingers of both hands, 36 times on each side. (Fig. 12-27)

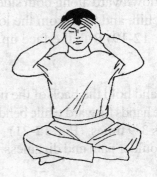

Fig. 12-18

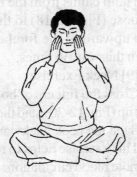

Fig. 12-19

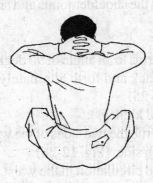

Fig. 12-20

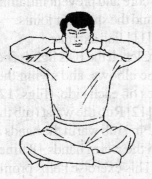

Fig. 12-21

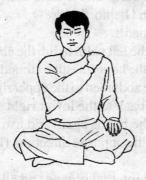

Fig. 12-22

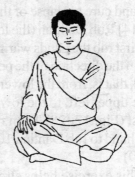

Fig. 12-23

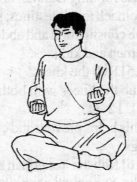

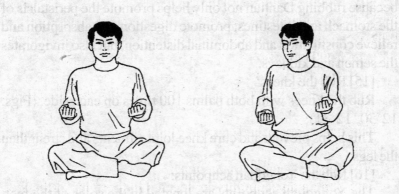

Fig. 12-24

Fig. 12-25

This exercise helps stimulate the nerves around the anus, improve their function, promote the local blood circulation, and prevent and cure prolapse of the rectum and hemorrhoids.

[14] Rub Dantian (the lower abdomen):

First rub the hands warm, then use the left palm to rub the abdomen in the direction of the peristalsis of the large intestine around the navel, that is, from the lower right of the abdomen to the upper right, to the upper left, to the lower left and back to the lower right 100 times. (Fig. 12- 28) Then rub warm the hands again and use the right hand to rub Dantian 100 times in the opposite direction. (Fig. 12-29)

This exercise helps strengthen the internal organs and adjust their functions.

If you suffer from emission, impotence or premature ejaculation, you might use one hand to cup the scrotum and use the other hand to rub Dantian. Rub it with either hand 81 times respectively. This is because rubbing Dantian not only helps promote the peristalsis of the stomach and intestines, promote digestion and absorption and relieve constipation and abdominal distention, but also invigorates the semen and kidneys.

[15] Rub the knees:

Rub the knees with both palms 100 times on each side. (Figs. 12-30, 12-31)

This helps prevent and cure knee joint ailments and strengthen the legs.

[16] Rub the Yongquan acupoints:

The Yongquan acupoints are located in the soles of the feet. First rub the right sole with the middle and index fingers of the left hand 100 times (Fig. 12-32), and then rub the left sole with the middle and index fingers of the right hand 100 times. (Fig. 12-33)

This exercise helps adjust the function of the heart and cures

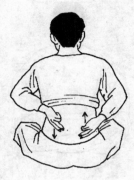

Fig. 12-26

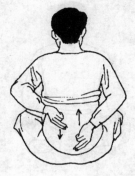

Fig. 12-27

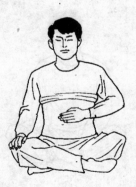

Fig. 12-28

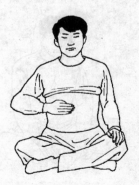

Fig. 12-29

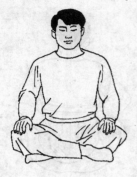

Fig. 12-30

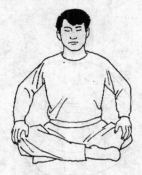

Fig. 12-31

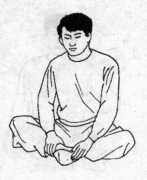

Fig. 12-32

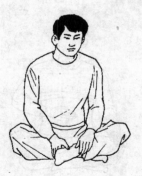

Fig. 12-33

dizziness.

[17] Weaving style:

Straighten the legs and keep them together, toes upward. Keep the palms outward in front of the chest and push them toward the feet. At the same time, bend the body forward and breathe out. Return after you push them to the end, but pull the palms inward and at the same time breathe in. (Figs. 12-34, 12-35) Repeat 30 times.

This exercise helps limber up the body to promote metabolism. It also has a special effect in preventing and curing lumbago and soreness of the loins.

[18] Mediate the belt vessel:

Sit naturally with crossed legs, hand in hand in front of the chest, and rotate the upper body from left to right 16 times and from right to left 16 times. Inhale while thrusting the chest (Fig. 12-36), and exhale while drawing the chest in. (Fig. 12-37)

This exercise helps strengthen the waist and kidneys, increase the movements of the stomach and intestines, and promote digestion and absorption.

(4) Walking exercise

The walking exercise is one of the dynamic exercises. While doing the walking exercise, couple it with breathing and mind concentration. You can do the whole set of exercises or choose some parts, depending on your physical condition.

The walking exercise consists of seven parts:

Starting form: Focus attention, keep quiet, relax your body, and stand erect with feet naturally apart at shoulder width. Draw the chest slightly in and keep the head upright, with the lower chin drawn in. Make sure that the head is not slanted and the scrotum is upright. Close the eyes slightly and look ahead with rapt attention. When you become calm, withdraw the look and keep the eyes on your

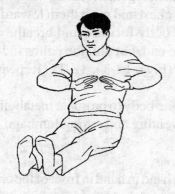

Fig. 12-34

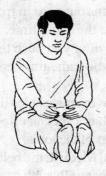

Fig. 12-35

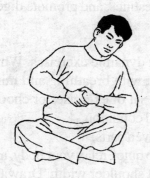

Fig. 12-36

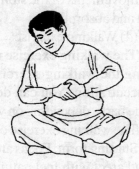

Fig. 12-37

own nose or close the eyes lightly and look internally at Dantian (the lower abdomen). Stick the tongue lightly against the upper palate without effort, and close the lips lightly or open them slightly, set the teeth lightly, drop the hands down naturally and breathe naturally. (Fig. 12-38)

[1] Get rid of the stale and take in the fresh:

When you begin the exercise, use the mind to guide the flow of the *qi* from Dantian to the arms and the hands. Move both palms from the sides outward, upward and inward to draw circles. When they are level with the head, cross the hands in front of the chest and then drop them to the abdomen. Do this 8-20 times. Inhale when raising the hands, and exhale when lowering the hands. Then, cross the hands in front of the lower abdomen, and move them upward, outward and downward. Inhale when raising the hands, and exhale when lowering the hands. Do this 8-20 times. (Fig. 12-39)

[2] Tap Dantian with fixed steps:

Clench the fists loosely, tap the Dantian region with the left fist, and tap the Mingmen (located at the back of the loins) with the back of the right palm. Coordinate it with breathing at the same time, and turn the waist simultaneously with the tapping. The tapping should be light, natural and relaxed. The number of taps should be identical with the number of breaths. Do it this way 10-30 times. (Figs. 12-40, 12-41)

After practising this exercise for some time, you may increase the range of waist turning and the range of hand swings so as to increase the activity of the spinal column and lumbar muscles. When you can do this very well, you may walk slowly while tapping for 5-10 minutes each time. (Fig. 12-42)

[3] Look at the hand form:

Use the mind to guide the flow of *qi* first to the left hand when the left palm is turned inward, and then move it from below upward and to the left outward. Keep both eyes on the left hand and follow the movement of the left hand, and move the right hand slowly from the right side to the abdomen. Drop the left hand slowly after it is raised to head level to the front left, and at the same time, move the right hand past the abdomen from below upward to the upper right outward. Move the hands alternately this way, and at the same time turn the waist. Inhale when raising the hand, and exhale when dropping the hand. Do this 10-30 times. (Fig. 12-43)

[4] Walking stake:

Concentrate the mind and stand erect, then squat down slightly, and shift the body weight to the right leg. Clench both fists simultaneously, coordinate it with breathing so as to circulate the qi to the feet. Raise the left foot a bit, toes touching the ground and the heel off the ground. After the *qi* flows down, move the left foot one step forward to the left, toes touching the ground. At the same time, change the fists into palms and push them forward, palms facing the front, left hand higher than the right hand, and eyes look at the left hand. While moving the left foot and pushing the palms, coordinate it with breathing. Relax the shoulders and elbows so they are comfortable and natural. Keep 70 percent of the weight on the right leg. (Figs. 12- 44, 12-45)

After moving the left foot forward, land the heel, and press the palms downward to the abdomen. When the body weight is shifted to the left leg, bend the left leg slightly and change both palms into fists. At the same time, touch the ground with the right toes, heels off the ground, and coordinate it with breathing. After standing firm, move the right foot one step forward to the right, toes on the ground. Change the fists into palms and press them forward to the right, and coordinate it with breathing. By this time, the right hand is higher than the left hand. Keep 70 percent of the weight on the left leg, and eyes look at the right hand. Keep on stepping forward along a

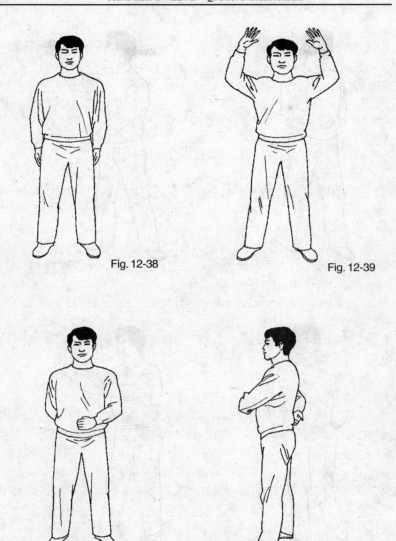

Fig. 12-38

Fig. 12-39

Fig. 12-40

Fig. 12-41

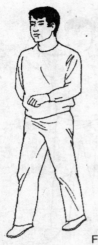

Fig. 12-42

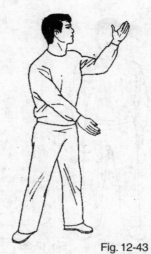

Fig. 12-43

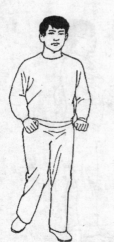

Fig. 12-44

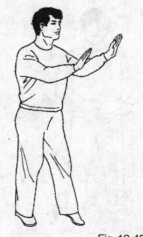

Fig. 12-45

straight line or around in a circle. The movements should be slow at the beginning, the rhythms clear, and the breathing properly coordinated. Practise it for 5 minutes at first, and gradually increase the time to 30 minutes, 2-4 times a day.

[5] Adjusting the balance:

Raise the arms to horizontal level on both sides, and at the same time raise the left leg, thigh at horizontal level and toes downward like a golden cock standing on one leg. Inhale while raising the arms, drop both arms while pausing, and land the left foot while exhaling. (Fig. 12-46) Then raise the arms to horizontal level on both sides, and at the same time raise the right leg with the ensuing movements the same as above. (Fig. 12-47)

Practise this exercise with fixed steps at the beginning and then practise the walking exercise. Move the feet forward step by step. Inhale while raising the leg and exhale while landing the foot. The hand movements are the same as in the fixed step exercise. You might walk straight ahead or around a circle.

[6] Kick the Changqiang acupoint with the heels:

Look ahead, breathe naturally and concentrate the mind on Dantian. When moving the right foot forward, throw the left leg backward energetically so that the heel touches the left buttock. Then move the left foot one step forward and throw the right leg backward energetically so that the heel touches the right buttock. (Figs. 12-48, 12-49)

Practise this exercise 2-4 times a day, and walk 50-100 steps each time.

[7] Rub horizontally around a Taiji circle:

First use the mind to guide the flow of *qi* from Dantian to the hands. Raise the hands slowly to navel level, palms downward and the radial sides of the hands opposite each other to form a Taiji circle. Relax the shoulders and drop the elbows so that the shoulders, elbows and wrists form a natural semicircle. Relax the hips, withdraw the buttocks, and bend the legs.

Then, rub with both hands horizontally to the left forward, the front and right forward around a circle. When moving both hands to the left forward, shift the body weight to the left leg, and move the right leg one step to the right side. When moving both hands to the front right, withdraw the left leg and keep the legs together. Rub this way 20 times, and then rub 20 times in the opposite direction. The movements should be soft and slow. (Figs. 12-50, 12-51)

The breathing method for this exercise:

Inhale when the hands are moved to the front left, and exhale when the hands are to the front of the abdomen. Attention: The air must be guided to Dantian, and it is better if you feel the lower abdomen filled with air. When exhaling, the lower abdomen must be drawn in. The breathing must be deep and long and the movements must be gentle and soft. Make sure that when in motion, the whole body moves, when in stillness, the whole body stops. There should be stillness in motion and motion in stillness.

(5) Ten-minute *qigong*

Many people are busy with work, study or household chore but still want to do some exercises though they do not have much time. Now we would like to recommend a set of *qigong* exercises which does not require much time or space. It generally takes only around 10 minutes. If you are very busy, just practise them for five minutes. If you have time, you may do them for 30 minutes.

In the beginning, it is best to practise this set of exercises in a quiet place. After you get used to it, you can do them even in a very noisy place.

Following is a description of the exercises:

[1] Posture: Standing, sitting and lying. Beginners do not have to pay much attention to the postures, just do them according to your

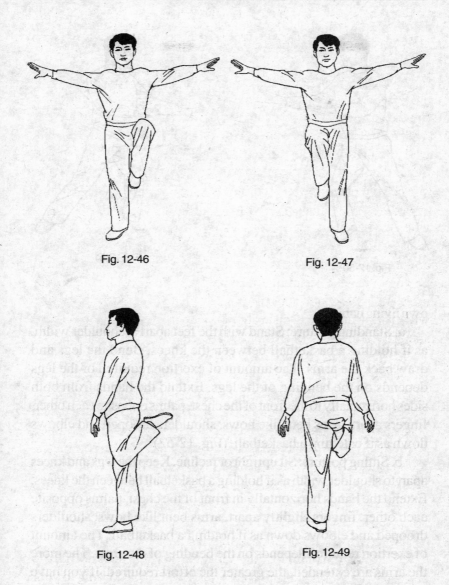

Fig. 12-46

Fig. 12-47

Fig. 12-48

Fig. 12-49

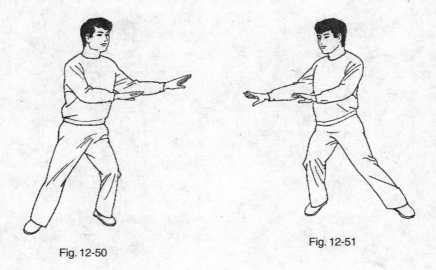

Fig. 12-50

Fig. 12-51

own living habits.

a. Standing posture: Stand with the feet apart at shoulder width, as if holding a basketball between the knees. Bend the legs and draw back the arms. The amount of exertion required of the legs depends on the bending of the legs. Extend the hands from both sides horizontally to the front of the chest, palms opposite each other, fingers apart, arms bent like bows, shoulders drooped and elbows down as if catching a basketball. (Fig. 12-52)

b. Sitting posture: Sit upright or recline. Keep the legs and knees apart to shoulder width as if holding a basketball between the knees. Extend the hands horizontally in front of the chest, palms opposite each other, fingers slightly apart, arms bent like bows, shoulders drooped and elbows down as if holding a basketball. The amount of exertion required depends on the bending of the arms. The more the arms are extended, the greater the effort required. If you have difficulty doing this, you can keep the upper arms vertical to form an angle of 90 degrees with the forearms, and extend the forearms horizontally forward. (Fig. 12-53)

c. Lying posture: Practising this exercise before sleep has a noticeable effect in curing insomnia. Raise the arms vertically upward, palms opposite each other and fingers slightly apart. Those with strong arms may also raise them obliquely, the arms forming an obtuse angle with the supine body, and the hands above the head. Keep the hands apart to shoulder width. If you find an abundant "sensation of *qi*" while practise *qigong*, you can extend both arms outward. The further apart the two hands are kept, the greater the amount of exertion required. (Fig. 12-54)

[2] Movements: Execute the opening and closing movements of both palms. Closed when the two palms are close to each other, and opened when the two palms are kept apart. The opening and closing movements of both knees can also be practised in sitting posture. The opening and closing movements are classified into four categories: large, small, slight and static. The opening and closing movements of the palms, and the holding together of the knees should be practised either separately or alternately to avoid diverting your attention.

[3] Mental activity: a. "Use the mind to recollect the opening and closing movements." This is the basic idea for practising *qigong* in the most effective way.

b. "Mental resistance." When doing the opening and closing movements, it is necessary to supplement them with mental resistance. That is, imagine there is a balloon, a spring or a rubber band with large resilience. They form the resistance to the opening and closing movements of the palms or knees. This mental resistance gives balanced exercise to the passages of the efferent nerve and the afferent nerve, the sensorium and the motor center. It is the basic condition

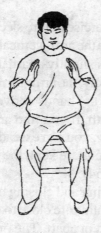

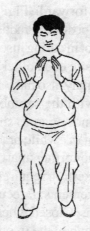

Fig. 12-53　　　　Fig. 12-52

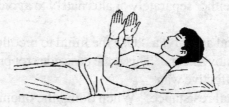

Fig. 12-54

for generating the "sensation of the *qi*," facilitating the circulation of the meridian energy, and removing obstructions in the channels and collaterals of the meridian system.

[4] Steps for practising *qigong*:

First execute the opening and closing movements. The frequency can be synchronous to the breathing with a large range of movement, or to the normal pulse with a small range of movement. Shift gradually from large opening and closing movements to slight opening and closing movements. At the same time, it is necessary to focus attention to the point where you are able to feel a slight motion. By this time, you will fall into quiescence naturally. Then turn to the opening and closing movements in stillness. That is, still in form, but with motion in the mind. That is motion in stillness.

In the course of practising *qigong*, physical movements and mental movements can be executed alternately, or they can permeate each other to take a varied form. When opening, the palms feel like magnets attracting or rubber bands pulling. This is called "closing in the opening." When closing, the palms feel like magnets repelling each other or like an air mass between the palms. They cannot close together. This is called "opening in the closing." Moreover, when executing a large opening movement, you can also execute some mental opening movements. It looks like motion, but it is not motion, and it looks like stopping, but it is not stopping. It is a combination of emptiness and solidity. When you execute the opening and closing of mental movements in stillness, as a result of the increased "sensation of *qi*" and its change, the palms open and close involuntarily. This is the combination of the mental movements and *qi*, and the use of *qi* to urge the motion.

[5] Indications and effect:

The 10-minute *qigong* helps to increase your mental ability to practise *qigong*, and improve your efficiency and memory in learning.

Beginners can start with the opening and closing of the palms, and then practise knee exercise when your experience of the "sensation of *qi*" is fully acquired.

People with dizziness or headache should not use their mind excessively, but they should mainly do the movements of opening and closing. Before sleep, they can practise the mental movements of opening and closing in the lying posture. When they get abundant "sensation of *qi*," they can put both palms slowly on the lower abdomen, and concentrate their mind on Dantian, namely, focus attention on the rise and fall, or the opening and closing of the Dantian region. This helps to cure insomnia and gastric and intestinal diseases.

People with palpitations might execute the movements of opening and closing as if holding a basketball between the knees to alleviate or even kill the symptom. Regular knee exercise helps to reduce the blood pressure and alleviate dizziness.

As long as you persevere in doing the 10-minute exercise, it is not difficult for you to learn to do it well.

(6) Sixteen-character formula exercise

[1] The 16-character formula exercise

The formula is: *yi xi bian ti* (while inhaling, raise the perineum), *qi qi sao qi* (all *qi* goes to the navel).

yi ti bian yan (while raising the perineum, swallow the saliva), *shui huo xiang jian* (The downgoing saliva meets the upflowing *qi*).

The exercise goes as follows:

a. Swallowing and inhaling: First rinse the mouth with saliva 3-5 times, keep on moving the tongue up and down, and stick the tongue against the upper palate to promote salivation. Swallow the saliva with gurgling sounds. Then immediately inhale a full breath through nose, use the mind to guide the swallowed saliva directly down to

Dantian. Hold it there for a while.

b. Raising and exhaling: Continue from the above movement, and raise the Huiyin (perineum) lightly as if holding back a bowel movement. At the same time, use the mind to guide the flow of *qi* upward to the navel, and raise it from the coccyx point and Jiaji acupoints on the back all way upward to the Yuzhen acupoint in the depression of the occiput and into the Niwan, an area behind the Yintang acupoint deep in the head. At the same time, put the tongue down lightly and exhale the stale air slowly.

Execute the movements of swallowing and inhaling, and raising and exhaling as described above alternately. Repeat the exercise, and swallow the saliva in 3-5 mouthfuls, or in 7-8 mouthfuls, or in 12 mouthfuls, or in 24 mouthfuls. Do what you want to do, and stop when you want to stop. But mind you, when you swallow the saliva, there must be gurgling sounds. The breathing should be long, fine and even. It is best that the ears not hearing any breath and for *qi* not to go out.

[2] The effect:

The 16-character *qigong* exercise helps to reinforce the primordial energy, promote digestion, remove obstructions in the channels and collaterals of the meridian system, and remove stasis. It is specially effective in curing diseases of the digestive system (gastritis, gastric ulcer, duodenal ulcer and ptosis of the stomach). It can also treat neurosis, hypertension, urinary incontinence, frequent micturition, excessive urination at night, hemorrhoids, anal fistula, and prolapse of the anus. As long as you persist in doing the exercises, you will find yourself vigorous, be sharp-sighted and sharp-eared, and free from illness.

[3] Health protection mechanism:

a. On swallowing the saliva: This exercise, first of all, helps produce more saliva in the mouth. The saliva, which was known as "golden fluid" in ancient times, is one of the five fluids in the human body, and is closely related to human life. Ancient physicians believed that "the tongue should be stuck against the palate, and the saliva should be frequently swallowed." They also said: "When you swallow it with gurgling sounds, all vessels are automatically balanced."

Therefore, frequent swallowing of saliva helps prevent and cure diseases in the alimentary canal.

b. On inhaling fresh air through the nose: The purpose of using the nose to draw fresh air and transmit it to Dantian is to obtain and replenish fresh air. The anion in the fresh air has a good effect in regulating the central nervous system, respiratory system, digestive system, circulatory system, blood-building system, and metabolism. Therefore, the frequent practise of inhaling fresh air through the nose has an inestimable effect in preserving good health and in preventing and curing diseases. It can improve the breathing function of the lungs, thus joining the internal organs in the control and regulation of the internal organs and the endocrine system.

c. On raising the Huiyin: Its purpose is to use the mind to guide the flow of *qi* (vital energy) upward to meet the saliva swallowed downward so that the water and the fire meet each other and the heart and kidneys communicate with each other. Perseverance in doing this exercise helps relieve dysentery and arrest seminal emission with astringents. It also has certain curative effects for dysentery, spermatorrhea, urinary incontinence, frequent micturition and excessive urination at night. Moreover, it helps to improve blood circulation and nutrition in the peripheral tissues of the anus, and helps prevent and cure hemorrhoids, anal fistula, and prolapse of the anus.

In short, this exercise is simple and easy to learn and has no side effects. It is not restricted by the surroundings, nor does it affect your study or work. As long as you are free any time of the day, you might as well do it.

(7) Sight-improving exercise

This is an exercise specially designed to improve the sight and train and protect the eyes.

[1] Procedure:

Either sit or stand. If you like to stand, keep the feet apart to the shoulder width and close the hands at Dantian. If you sit, sit upright, put the hands in front of the forehead, and keep the body relaxed and the mind quiet. When practising this exercise, execute the movements quickly at first and then slowly, and direct the flow of *qi* and blood evenly and silently.

[2] Methods:

This exercise consists of four methods: the method of directing *qi* through the liver meridian, the method of sight improvement, the method of directing *qi* at fixed points, and the method of directing *qi* by pressing the acupoints around the eyes.

a. The method of directing *qi* through the liver meridian: This is a method for curing diseases by directing *qi* through the liver meridian. Both the posture and points for attention are the same as described above. Close the eyes, relax the body, use the mind to guide the flow of *qi* through the liver meridian, starting from the Dadun acupoints (located on the lateral sides of the big toes), along the shanks, the inner sides of the thighs into the abdomen, upward to the Qimen acupoints on the chest, and then through the throat upward to the eyes. Open the eyes, look at a fixed target several meters ahead, and imagine the removal of the stale *qi* from inside the eyes. Practise this repeatedly. (Fig. 12-55)

b. The method of sight improvement: This is a method of directing *qi* around the eyes to improve the sight. The posture and points for attention are the same as described above. Close the eyes, relax the body, and concentrate the mind. First close the eyes to look internally, then look up and down, to the right, to the left, and ahead. And then look by turning the eyes first from left to right, and then from right to left. Practise this repeatedly. (Figs. 12-56, 12-57, 12-58)

c. The method of directing *qi* at fixed points: This refers to the selection of a certain fixed point for the direction of *qi*. The posture and points for attention are the same as described above. Close the eyes, relax the body, and concentrate the mind. Then look at a selected point in the distance several meters away, perhaps a tree or a flowering plant. Open the eyes wide and glare like a tiger. Then close the eyes to look internally. Then open one eye and close the other. Practise repeatedly. (Figs. 12-59, 12-60)

d. The method of directing *qi* by pressing the meridian points around the eyes: This is a method for directing *qi* to the fingers and using the mind to point and press the meridian points around the eyes. The posture and points for attention are the same as described above. Close the eyes, relax the body, concentrate the mind and use the mind to guide the flow of *qi* to the index and middle fingers to press the meridian points, starting from Baihui, along the Du channel, past the Shenting into Yintang acupoints (the route is Baihui-Shenting-Yintang, Fig. 12-61). Then, press the acupoints around the eyes, along the route of Yintang-Zanzhu-Yanmei (Yuyao)-Sizhukong, the eye corner (Tongziliao)-Qiuhou-Chengqi-Jianming-Jingming. First press from the bow of the left eyebrow to the bow of the right eyebrow, and then from below the right eye socket to the left eye socket. Press around the circle clockwise and counterclockwise seven times respectively. (Fig. 12-62) Finally, press from Baihui-Yintang, along the separate routes from the left and right eyebrows around the eyes, past Jingming acupoints downward to the Yingxiang acupoints on the two sides of the nose to join at the Renzhong acupoint. The *qi* flows from the chest down to Dantian. Practise this

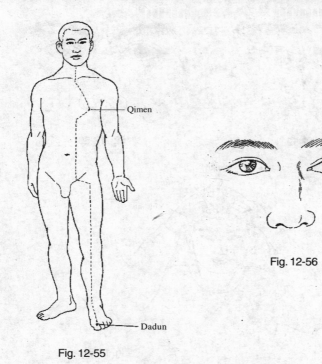

Fig. 12-55

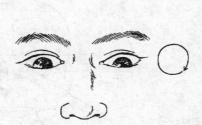

Fig. 12-56

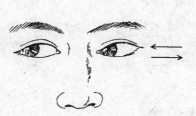

Fig. 12-57

Fig. 12-58

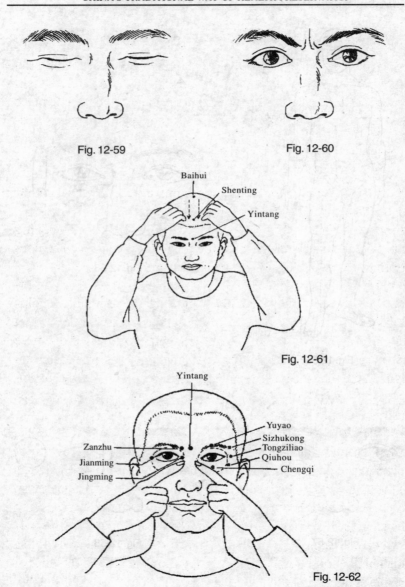

Fig. 12-59

Fig. 12-60

Fig. 12-61

Fig. 12-62

way repeatedly.

[3] Closing form:

Raise both hands slowly upward to shoulder level, bend the elbows, fingers pointing at each other, palms downward. Press them downward lightly by both sides. Or put the palms together and place the right hand on top of the left hand (women in the opposite direction) pressing against Dantian in the lower abdomen. Close the eyes for a few seconds to close the form. (Fig. 12-63)

[4] Mind concentration and breathing

Fall into quiescence through the adjustment of mental activities, breathe naturally, close the eyes to maintain normal breathing, smooth the eyebrows and expand the chest. Inhale while opening the eyes, and exhale while closing the eyes. Coordinate mind concentration with breathing while practising this exercise.

[5] Indications: The exercise is simple and easy to learn. Its effect will be seen after practising it for one or two months. It helps improve the function of the eyes, adjust the cerebral nerve, correct and improve the eye sight of young people, and has a preventive and curative effect for declining sight, myopia, weak sight, astigmatism and farsightedness. It also helps to strengthen the brains, improve fitness, and has a certain effect in relieving headache, neurosis, insomnia and liver diseases.

[6] Effect:

a. Reaction from the sensation of *qi*: You may feel warm or relaxed around the eyes when practising the exercise or shed tears at the beginning. Both are normal reactions, so do not mind them.

b. Bad reaction: Just reduce the number of times you practising the exercise if you have dim sight or shed tears after doing it for 1-3 weeks. Avoid exerting too much effort. Breathe slowly. It is a normal phenomenon if you see red, yellow, green, blue, white or purple spots or rings.

[7] Time and number of repititions:

Practise once or twice a day, 15-20 minutes each time. Once for each form, and 7-21 repititions each session.

(8) Static *qigong* exereise for the prevention and treatment of myopia

The advantages of static *qigong* are: It is easy to learn and practise, safe and reliable, and has a good curative effect for young people, children, and adults suffering from myopia.

The exercise consists of three parts: Standing still for *qi* preservation, directing *qi* with opening and closing movements, and massaging the eyes with the external *qi*. The first two are the basics.

[1] Stand still for *qi* preservation:

Posture: Similar to standing at attention, legs together, feet apart, about a fist's space between the big toes.

Relax the knees, put the body weight on the soles, feet flat on the ground.

Tuck in the hips and do not thrust them forward.

Draw in the buttocks so they do not protrude.

Keep the spinal column straight, relax the waist, flatten the chest, relax the abdomen, and keep the body upright.

Keep the head upright, neck straight, withdraw the forehead, hide the larynx, and keep the tip of the nose in vertical line with the navel, relax the eyelids, close the eyes slightly, breathe naturally, close the mouth slightly, and stick the tongue against the upper palate.

Relax the shoulders, both arms down naturally, fingers by the seams of the trousers, back of the hands obliquely forward, the fingers apart loosely, palms open, middle fingers naturally extended, and arms relaxed. (Fig. 12-64)

In the still standing *qigong* exercise, you should keep your head upright, body erect, feet flat and arms stretched, so that the movements of the upper and lower limbs are well coordinated, the entire body relaxed, and the mind concentrated. Do it for 15 minutes each session.

[2] Directing *qi* with opening and closing movements

Posture: While standing still, keep the toes of both feet together. Move the left foot to the left and keep the feet apart at shoulder width.

Move both hands slowly upward to shoulder level. (Fig. 12-65)

Bend the knees slightly to a sitting stance. At the same time, relax the shoulders and drop the elbows to bend the arms into semi-circles, wrists at shoulder level and palms facing each other. Make sure that the Laogong acupoints in the center of the palms are opposite each other and are inter-connected. (Fig. 12-66)

Relax the hands, and when both palms feel slightly numb and warm, close the hands slowly inward as if pressing a balloon between them until they are 6-7 cm apart, and then pull them slowly outward to shoulder width. Then close the hands slowly again. Repeat the pulling and closing movements for 5 minutes until you feel you can no longer pull them apart or close them, or they close and open automatically. (Figs. 12-67, 12-68)

This exercise enables the intrinsic *qi* and outgoing *qi* to respond to each other. It not only helps regulate the flow of *qi* through the channels to improve the functions of the internal organs, but also brings the external *qi* under the control of your mind to treat myopia.

[3] Massage the eyes with the external *qi*.

Take off your glasses when you practise this exercise.

The exercise consists of five sections:

a. When you find the sensation of *qi* in your hands very strong while directing *qi* with opening and closing movements, turn the hands slowly over so that the Laogong acupoints in the center of the palms face both eyes. Hold the *qi* in the palms and bring them slowly close

ments of the upper and lower limbs are well coordinated, the entire body relaxed and the mind concentrated. Do it for 15 minutes each session.

[2] Exercising with open eyes and moving canvas.

Posture: Sit or stand in such a position that the line of sight moves from left to right and forth and back. Keep apart at shoulder width.

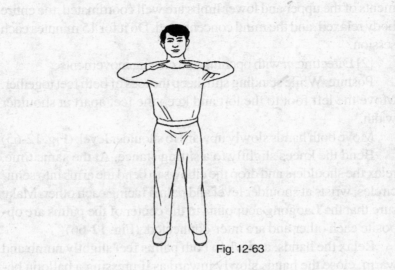

Fig. 12-63

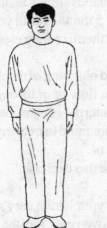

Fig. 12-64

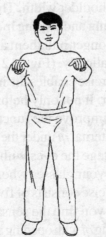

Fig. 12-65

in the eyes until they ache (Fig. 12-71) or away, and the eyes feel pressure or cool warmth. Practice this for one minute so that the heat of the palms penetrates into the eyeballs and joins the *qi* in the eyeballs (Figs. 12-69 & 12-70).

6. When both of your hands join the *qi* in the eyeballs, pull the palms slowly out to about 30 centimeter the eyes. This moves the *qi* slowly into the eyeballs until the palms are 6 inches the eyes. Then pull and push slowly. Repeat this way three times (Figs. 12-71, 12-72A, 72B, and keep the palms at about 1 foot from the eyes. When pulling and pressing, find a feeling of attraction and repulsion between the hands and the eyes. The feeling differs from person to person.

7. Keep the palms and the eyes at the same distance. While maintaining a link between the hands and the eyes, circle slowly with both hands in the same direction, first to the left and then to the right, 3–6 times in each direction. The circles should not be too large. Use the *qi* in the hands to drive the *qi* in the eyes to produce a feeling of rotation (Fig. 12-73).

8. Stop in place after turning, and let the palms oppose the eyeballs. Move your body with the arms and circulate the *qi* in the palms to massage the eyeballs, nourishing eyesight and improving blood circulation. The massage takes about 3 minutes (Fig. 12-74).

9. Winding the eyes anew. Move the hands slowly toward the eyes through a small circle. After a pause of about 1 minute, rub the eyes with both hands in the same direction, to the left, and then to the right, 3–6 times in each direction. (Figs. 12-75, 12-76). After a slight pause, stroke down your face with both hands as though washing the face from the forehead downward to the two inner corners of the eyes, along the sides of the nose to the chest and abdomen (Fig. 12-77). Feel rejuvenated. At the same time, keep your

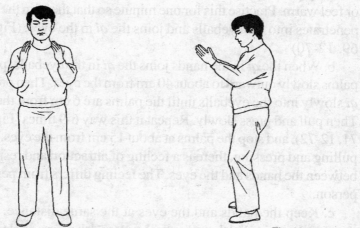
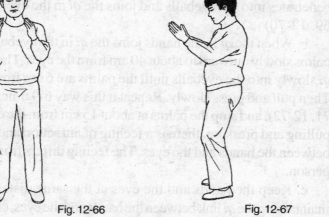

Fig. 12-66

Fig. 12-67

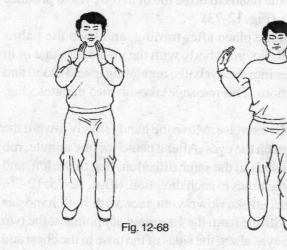
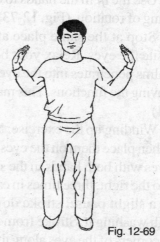

Fig. 12-68

Fig. 12-69

331

to the eyes until they are 6-12 cm away and the eyes feel pressure or feel warm. Practise this for one minute so that the *qi* in the palms penetrates into the eyeballs and joins the *qi* in the eyes. (Figs. 12-69, 12-70)

b. When the *qi* in the hands joins the *qi* in the eyeballs, pull the palms slowly outward to about 40 cm from the eyes. Then press the *qi* slowly into the eyeballs until the palms are 6 cm from the eyes. Then pull and press slowly. Repeat it this way 6-9 times (Figs. 12-71, 12-72), and stop the palms at about 15 cm from the eyes. When pulling and pressing, there is a feeling of attraction and resistance between the hands and the eyes. The feeling differs from person to person.

c. Keep the hands and the eyes at the same distance. While maintaining the *qi* link between the hands and the eyes, circle slowly with both hands in the same direction, first to the left and then to the right, 3-6 times in each direction. The circles should not be too large. Use the *qi* in the hands to drive the *qi* in the eyes to produce a feeling of rotation. (Fig. 12-73)

d. Stop at the same place after turning, and keep the palms opposite the eyes. Relax your body with the awareness that *qi* in the palms penetrates into the eyeballs, regulating *qi* and blood and improving the functions. This massage takes about 5 minutes. (Fig. 12-74)

e. Winding up the exercise: Move the hands slowly toward the eyes then place them on the eyes. After a pause for one minute, rub the eyes with both hands in the same direction, first to the left, and then to the right, three times in each direction. (Figs. 12-75, 12-76) After a slight pause, stroke down your face with both hands as though washing it. Stroke from the Jingming acupoints at the two inner corners of the eyes along the sides of the nose to the chest and abdomen (Fig. 12-77), feet together. At the same time, keep your

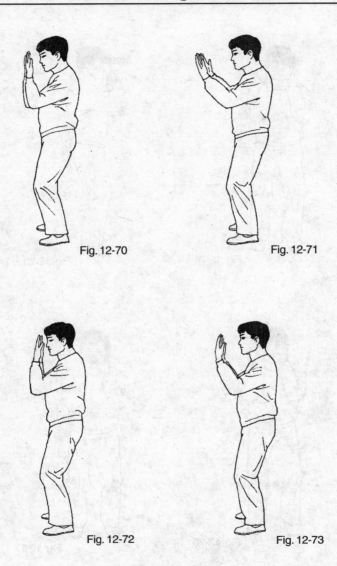

Fig. 12-70

Fig. 12-71

Fig. 12-72

Fig. 12-73

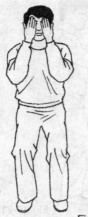

Fig. 12-74

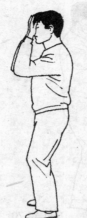

Fig. 12-75

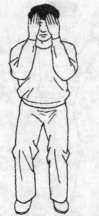

Fig. 12-76

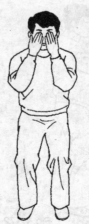

Fig. 12-77

hands by your sides and return to the standing still position. After standing for a while, open the eyes slowly, look to the left, look to the right, then look to the distance to get a clear sight.

It takes about 30 minutes to finish this whole set of exercises, two sessions a day, one in the morning and one in the evening.

Practice is not restricted by time. You can do it any time of day, before meals, after meals, in the morning, in the evening, during work breaks or between classes. First, stand still for 2-3 minutes, and then do the *qi* directing exercise and eye massage for 5-10 minutes. Beginners should spend more time on the *qi* directing exercise, not less than 5 minutes each time. If you feel a strong sensation of *qi* as soon as you close your hands, you can turn to doing more eye massage. At first, you can consolidate the curative effect only by persisting in doing the exercise for three months or longer. At the same time, take care of your eyes because even if you get good results from practising the exercise, it is very difficult to consolidate it.

(9) Mental training exercise

The mental training exercise is a method of treating illness and improving fitness by controlling mental activities through mind concentration and the control of desires.

All *qigong* exercises stress mental training, and there is no *qigong* that does not stress mental training. However, there are some differences between this exercise and other *qigong* exercises.

[1] Posture: Standing, sitting and lying.

a. Standing posture: Stand erect, with feet apart to shoulder width, head upright, eyes ahead, and slightly closed, and chin slightly drawn in. Draw in the chest, droop the shoulders, contract the abdomen, and bend the knees slightly. The buttocks are in a sitting position, but are not actually sitting. Raise both arms forward, palms downward, not higher than eyebrows, nor lower than navel, about 33 cm to the body. Keep the fingers apart, fingertips slightly inward.

b. Sitting posture: Sit erect on a stool without leaning backward. Keep the upper body in the same position as in the standing posture, with the feet and legs apart to shoulder width. Lower the shanks naturally and bend the knees to form a right angle, feet flat on the ground.

c. Lying posture: Lying on the back or lying on the side.

d. Lying on the back: Lying supine on a bed, keep the upper part of the body in the same position as in the standing posture, legs straight and palms upward

e. Lying on the side: Lying either on the left or right side, the lower leg straight and the upper leg slightly bent. Put the upper hand on the thigh, palm downward, and the lower hand on the pillow, palm upward.

The choice of a posture depends on the individual. Start the mental exercises right after taking the posture.

[2] Mental exercises:

There are two kinds of mental exercises: One is for the beginners and the other is for those who have been practising for a long time. There is a difference between the two.

At the start, mental exercises should be conducted in the following order:

a. Throw a ball: Take a high mountain, a big river, a pavilion, an ancient tower or even the blue sky as your target and then imagine you have thrown a ball, your mind and body were also thrown out with the ball, and returned with the ball after reaching the target. Go and return, loosen and tighten. Just keep on throwing the ball and returning like this, and you find your body becomes comfortable and soothed, the *qi* and blood flowing without obstruction.

b. Embrace a mountain: Imagine your arms and hands are embracing a high mountain or a large tower in the distance. Imagine that your own body is becoming larger and larger, until it becomes large enough to hold the mountain or tower in your arms. Embrace it and let it go, loosen and tighten. Do it repeatedly like this.

c. Lift the head upward: Imagine there is a hanging rope at the Baihui acupoint on the top of your head and it extends far into the blue sky. And imagine that your whole body is being lifted up and landed down by the blue sky and all the internal organs are also rising and falling with your body. Mind you, the rise and fall start from the Baihui acupoint. This exercise is practised entirely through your imagination.

If you feel relaxed, pleasant and comfortable after ball-throwing, mountain-embracing and head-lifting exercise, you have succeeded in this training exercise. After practising for 3-6 months, your body and all its internal organs will relax or tighten at a hint from your imagination. As a result of this relaxation, your nervous and internal systems will be regulated and strengthened. If you feel a pain, a quiver, or warmth in the affected region when the internal organs are relaxed, this is a good sign. Do not worry or stop practising. Hypertension sufferers should not do the head-lifting exercises.

After practising ball-throwing, mountain-embracing and head-lifting exercises for 6-12 months, you can begin doing the following exercises:

a. Three holds and two butts: The three holds are: Imagine you are holding balls between your knees, thighs and the ankles. The two butts are: Imagine there is a target in the distance, and butt the target with your toes and knees, and a rubber band keeps pulling and loosening between your toes and knees and the target.

b. Bulge the waist and pull the back: Imagine you are bulging your waist out like a gourd and pulling your back upward. All these are imaginary movements, and the waist and back do not move at all. This exercise helps train both the waist and the back.

c. Look like you are sitting, but do not sit, and look like your neck and collar stuck together, but they are not: Imagine you are seated, but without a stool or a chair. Imagine your neck sticks to the collar, but it actually does not. Both movements are imaginary.

There is a greater degree of difficulty in practising these three exercises, but they produce good curative effects for some chronic diseases. You should have acquired some basics before beginning these exercises, and it also requires long-time perseverance. After you practise it for a long time, you will find yourself in a state of complete adaptation of the human body to the environment, namely, the so-called "complete unity of the human body and the natural environment."

This exercise is good for all those suffering from chronic diseases, especially those who are confined to bed and cannot participate in other activities. It also helps the healthy improve their physical fitness.

[3] Points for attention:

a. Do the exercise in a quiet place with fresh air. It does not do any good to practise on windy or rainy days or in the sweltering summer or freezing winter.

b. The best time to do it is early in the morning, for 30-60 minutes. This can be shorter for the beginners and can be extended as your skill improves. Physically weak people and the ill should practise for only 3-10 minutes a time, 1-3 times a day.

c. In general, it is best to take the standing posture, but the older, physically weak and sick people may sit or lie down. Do the standing exercise outdoors and the sitting or lying exercise indoors.

d. Unbutton your clothes, adjust your breathing, concentrate your mind, and keep yourself relaxed and calm before exercising.

e. You will often find some unusual feelings after doing the exercise, such as hallucinations. Sometimes there emerges an illusory ray of light before your eyes, the place where you stand seems to be rocking, your body seems to become smaller or larger, the limbs shorter or longer, the waist swelling, the head rising against the sky. Do not be alarmed. This is the reflection of the mental exercises. It you open your eyes, the hallucinations will disappear immediately.

There might be some other unusual feelings. For example, you may feel warm, or your body itches, or sometimes your body shakes, you hiccup or break wind. These are signs of the smooh circulation of blood and the improved function of the internal organs. Do not be alarmed. They disappear as soon as you finish the exercise.

Sometimes, there is an internal appearance. That is, as you practise, it seems that you can hear the sounds of the flow of blood through the body, or can see your own internal organs. This demonstrates that you have acquired perfect skills in the exercises. Be neither alarmed nor too elated.

(10) Kidney-lifting exercise

The kidney-lifting exercise is one in which you concentrate the mind on the perineum. Lift the private parts up and down and contract the privates upward and inward while breathing, as if holding back urination. This is one of the *qigong* exercises, and it is done like this:

[1] Sit upright on a stool with the feet on the ground and apart to shoulder width. Put the hands on the thighs, palms either up or down. Sit only partially, not completely, on the stool. When you have acquired good skill in this exercise, you may do it freely, any time and any place you like, without confining yourself to any particular form.

[2] Concentrate the mind on the perineum and dispel all distracting thoughts. While you breathe, contract the private parts inward by lifting them up and letting go as if holding back urination.

[3] Use the abdominal breathing method, that is, contract the abdomen while inhaling. At the same time, exert some effort to lift

the private parts upward. Relax the abdomen and let go the private parts while exhaling. Lift the private parts up and let go while breathing, and repeat it. Do the exercise 1-3 times every day, and lift and contract the private parts 10-20 times each exercise.

The private parts refer to the anus and the genitals.

Indications:

This exercise is good for many chronic diseases, particularly emission, premature ejaculation, cystitis, adrenal tuberculosis, prostatitis, enterogastritis, hematuria, metroptosis, prolapse of the anus, chronic diarrhoea, neurosis, regenerative anemia, and hypertrophic spondylitis. The curative effect is even better in treating diseases in the urogenital system.

Contraindications:

There are no absolute contraindications for this exercise. However, practitioners should properly control the amount of physical exertion, depending on their own condition. For example, hypertension sufferers should decrease the number of times they lift and contract the private parts each session to guard against dizziness and rising blood pressure. Insomniaes should not practise *qigong* in the evening.

Points for attention:

[1] Both men and women can practise this exercise.

[2] Do not contract or lift the private parts more than 20 times each session or it will cause tension at the top of the head.

[3] Do not practise the exercise when you are tired, angry, hungry or in a bad mood. Stop doing the exercise when you feel your head swimming.

(11) Eight-section brocade *qigong* exercise

The eight-section brocade *qigong* exercise is a dynamic exercise offering the dual advantages of *qigong* and health preservation. It consists of the eight-section brocade exercise for health protection created 800 years ago, the adjustment of breathing, and the adjustment of mental activities.

This exercise is simple and easy to learn and the amount of physical exertion required can be either great or small depending on the individual. You may practise the entire set, or choose as many sections as you like.

This exercise can strengthen the limbs, develop the thoracic muscles, improve health and beauty, prevent curvature of the spinal column, and prevent and cure some common chronic diseases such as cervical vertebra disorder, lumbago, sore legs, and stomachache. And perseverance may add years to your life.

It can be practised either early in the morning or in the evening, in a place with fresh air and pleasant surroundings. It will take 15-30 minutes a day.

The eight sections are:

[1] Hold up the sky with both hands to regulate the triple energizer

a. Starting position: Stand with the feet parallel to each other, arms naturally down, and look ahead.

b. Essential points: Raise the arms slowly upward from both sides, and at the same time cross the fingers and turn the palms upward, fingers opposite each other. Straighten the arms energetically as if holding up the sky. At the same time, raise the head and look up at the hands, throw out the chest, contract the abdomen, and straighten the back. Then put the arms and hands down slowly on both sides. Alternately raise and put down the arms in this way. (Fig. 12-78)

c. Mental activity and breathing: Use the mind to guide the flow of *qi* to rise and fall, and *qi* flows together with the warmth. Regulated by your consciousness, inhale while turning the palms upward to hold up the sky, and exhale while dropping both hands to the sides of the body. Do this repeatedly.

d. Indications and effect: This helps build up the body gracefully, reduce weight, prevent hunchback, strengthen the muscles in the chest, enlarge the range of activity in the thoracic cavity, improve breathing, and the function of the spinal column, and prevent cervical vertebra disease, inflammation around the shoulders and spinal curvature.

[2] Draw bows on both sides as if shooting at a vulture

a. Starting position: Stand with the feet parallel and apart to shoulder width, and the arms down naturally, and look ahead.

b. Essential points: Move the left foot one step to the left to form the horse-riding stance. Keep the upper body upright with the arms crossed in front of the chest, left arm inside and right arm outside, and fingers apart. First push with the right hand to the right and at the same time change the left hand into a claw-like fist and pull it to the left as if pulling a giant bow until the right arm is fully extended with the left elbow stretching to the left side. Look at the right hand, then change direction, with the left hand pushing to the left and the right hand pulling the bow to the right side. Do this exercise from both directions alternately.

c. Mental activity and breathing: Use the mind to guide the flow of *qi* to the outward pushing hand. Inhale while drawing the bow, and exhale while withdrawing the hands.

d. Indications and effect: This exercise is used mainly to prevent and treat cervical and shoulder disorders, lumbago, sore legs, osteomalacia of the kneecaps, and hyperplasia of the bones.

[3] Regulate the spleen and stomach with one arm raised

a. Starting position: Stand with the feet parallel and the arms down naturally, and look ahead.

b. Essential points: Raise the right hand upward on the right side, with the palm turned upward, fingers together. Straighten the right arm forcefully, palm upward, fingertips toward the left. At the same time, press downward forcefully with the left palm, fingertips forward. Then, raise the left hand upward on the left side, with the palm turned upward, fingers together. Straighten the left arm energetically, palm upward, fingertips toward the right. At the same time, drop the right hand on the right side, and press the palm downward, fingertips forward. Do the exercise this way alternately. (Fig. 12-80)

c. Mental activity and breathing: Use the mind to guide the flow of the *qi* along with the stance changes. Receive the Yang *qi* when the hand raises, and release the stale air when the hand is pressing downward. Inhale when raising and pressing the hand, and exhale when withdrawing the arms.

d. Indications and effect: This is used mainly to regulate the function of the spleen and stomach, and prevent and cure diseases of the digestive system, shoulder ailments and weakness in the arms.

[4] Look back to relieve five strains and seven injuries

a. Starting position: Stand erect with feet forward, the neck erect, arms down naturally and palms against the sides of the thighs.

b. Essential points: Throw out the chest, draw the shoulders slightly backward. At the same time, turn the head slowly to the left and look backward. Return to the original posture. Then turn the head slowly to the right and look backward. Do this exercise repeatedly in opposite directions. (Fig. 12-81)

c. Mental activity and breathing: Use the abdominal breathing. Inhale while looking backward, and exhale when returning to the original posture. Concentrate the mind on Dantian.

d. Indication and effect: This is used mainly to prevent and cure diseases of the cervical vertebra.

[5] Shake the head and wag the tail to remove heart-fire

a. Starting position: Stand with feet apart, wider than shoulder width. Bend the knees to form the horse-riding stance. Put hands

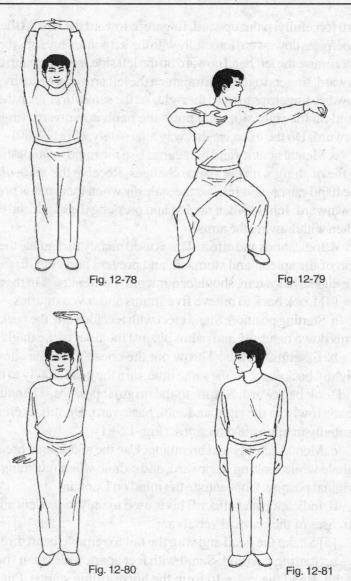

Fig. 12-78

Fig. 12-79

Fig. 12-80

Fig. 12-81

on knees with the radial sides inward. Keep the upper body upright.

b. Essential points: Bend the upper body deeply to the left, lower the head, swing it to the right, and shake it. Swing the buttocks slightly to the left, and then return to the starting position. Then bend the upper body forward deeply to the right, lower the head, swing it to the left, and shake it. At the same time, swing the buttocks slightly to the right and then return to the original position. Do the exercise in both directions alternately. (Fig. 12-82)

c. Mental activity and breathing: Concentrate the mind on Dantian, and breathe naturally.

d. Indications and effect: This is used mainly to prevent and treat neurosis, irritability and restlessness. It helps relieve mental strain and improve the functions of the waist and knee joints.

[6] Hold the feet with both hands to strengthen the kidney and waist

a. Starting position: Stand erect with feet apart and relax.

b. Essential points: Bend the upper body slowly forward and downward, and keep the knees as straight as possible. At the same time, drop the arms downward, hands touching the toes, and look at the hands. Then do a back-stretching exercise by putting the hands on either the Shenshu or Mingmen acupoint and bending the upper body gradually backward until you can stand firm. Bend the body forward and backward alternately. (Fig. 12-83, 12-84)

c. Mental activity and breathing: Use the mind to guide the flow of the *qi* along with the movements of the hands. Exhale while bending the body forward and inhale while bending the body backward. Concentrate the mind on inhaling and direct the *qi* into the back part of Dantian to strengthen the waist and kidneys.

d. Indications and effect: This is used mainly to strengthen the functions of the waist and kidneys and is also good for lumbago sufferers.

[7] Clench fists with angry eyes to increase physical strength

a. Starting position: Stand with the feet apart, and bend the knees to form the horse-riding stance. Clench the fists and place them by the sides, with fists facing up.

b. Essential points: Thrust the right fist forward slowly with consciousness, stretch the arm with the fist facing down. At the same time, clench the left fist tightly and thrust the left elbow backward. Open the eyes wide to stare forward, then withdraw the right fist to the side. Then thrust the left fist slowly forward with consciousness, and at the same time clench the right fist tightly with the right elbow thrust backward. Open your eyes wide and stare forward. Return to the original position. Repeat the exercise alternately. (Fig. 12-85)

c. Mental activity and breathing: Transform the mental consciousness into strength, and use the mind to increase strength when thrusting the fists. Inhale while thrusting the fists, and exhale while withdrawing the hands. Flow *qi* into the middle part of Dantian to conserve *qi* and promote strength.

d. Indications and effect: This is used to prevent and treat ailments of the neck, shoulder and waist, and for strengthening the entire body.

[8] Jolt backward seven times to cure all diseases

a. Starting position: Stand erect and relax the body, feet together, and palms against the thighs.

b. Essential points: Thrust the chest forward and straighten the legs. Raise the head upward as much as possible. At the same time, raise the heels as much as possible. Then land the heels and return to the original position. Raise and land the heels seven times alternately. (Fig. 12-86)

c. Mental activity and breathing: Use the mind to guide the flow of *qi* along with the movements of the body. Inhale when raising the

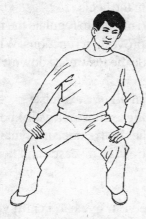

Fig. 12-82

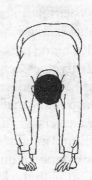

Fig. 12-83

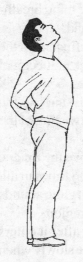

Fig. 12-84

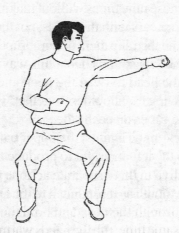

Fig. 12-85

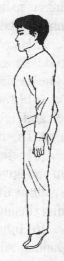

Fig. 12-86

head and heels, and exhale when landing the heels.

d. Indications and effect: This is used mainly to regulate the meridian system and internal organs and improve their functions. While doing this exercise, use the mind to guide the flow of *qi* downward to reduce blood pressure..

(12) Twelve-section brocade internal *qigong* exercise

The 12-section brocade internal *qigong* exercise is a well-known physical training method which combines both static and dynamic *qigong* exercises. This exercise helps treat all diseases and keeps the body and mind sound and healthy.

The exercise is done like this:

[1] Sit with the legs crossed, close your eyes and calm your mind. Hold the thumbs in the fingers, and hold your breath to preserve vitality.

[2] Click the upper and lower teeth 36 times, and then cross the fingers to hold the back of the head, and count in your mind breathing through the nose nine times without making a sound.

[3] Cover your ears with the hands, put the index fingers on the middle fingers and then slip them down abruptly to flick the occipital bones with a cracking sounds. Do it this way 24 times.

[4] Lower the head to twist the neck and look askance to the left and right. Swing the shoulders together with the twisting of the neck. Do this 24 times on each side.

[5] Stick the tongue against the upper palate, move the tongue up and down to the left and right to produce saliva, 36 times in all. Swallow the saliva in three separate actions with gurgling sounds after rinsing the mouth as if sending it to the Dantian region.

[6] Inhale through the nose and hold the breath after it enters Dantian. At the same time, rub the hands warm. Exhale slowly when massaging the back side of the waist with the warm hands. Do this 36 times before withdrawing the hands and clenching the fists tightly.

[7] Hold the breath and imagine that the fire in the heart is burned down to Dantian. When you feel warm, discharge the *qi* slowly and must not let the *qi* stop at Dantian.

[8] Bend the elbows and shake the arms. Move the arms in a circle with the shoulders as the axis, as if operating a winch, first to the left and then to the right. Do this 36 times.

[9] Stretch the feet, cross the hands and turn the palms upward. First press the top of the head and then hold it upward forcefully as if lifting something heavy. At the same time, raise the upper body upward forcefully. Repeat it 9 times.

[10] Bend your head forward and stretch the hands to grab the feet as if bowing in a religious service. Repeat the exercise 12 times. Then withdraw the feet, sit up straight, and clench the fists.

[11] Repeat rinsing the mouth with saliva exercise three times, and swallow the saliva in three actions each time. Swallow the saliva with gurgling sounds 9 times in all to regulate the pulse.

[12] Concentrate the mind on Dantian below the navel as if the warmth is burning like fire. Then transmit it to the anus and then raise it to the waist and back, and finally to the top of the head through the neck and the back of the head. Then lower it from the temples, before the roots of the ears, past the cheeks down to the throat, through the breasts and to Dantian. When the whole body feels warm, wind up the exercise.

The best time for doing this exercise is between 23:00-1:00 or between 11:00-13:00.

(13) Six-character formula

The six-character formula, consisting of the six Chinese characters "*xu-he- hu-si-chui-xi*," was a method of preserving health in ancient China. The six Chinese characters are used while breathing out to remove obstructions in the channels and collaterals of the meridian system and regulate the flow of *qi* and blood in the internal organs to improve health and treat diseases.

Since it is simple and easy to learn, it has always been very popular among the people. It has a wonderful effect in treating some chronic conditions such as coronary heart disease, hypertension, hypotension, hepatitis, enterogastritis, bronchitis, diabetes, neurosis, ossification, and even some cancers.

This is an abdominal breathing method for producing sounds while exhaling, by reading the six characters in order: *xu, he, hu, si, chui* and *xi*. All these sounds are uttered in the first tone, i.e., high and flat and cut off only when the utterer wishes. It only requies 30 minutes of practice everyday.

The exercise is done in this way:

Starting form:

Dispel distracting thoughts and keep both body and mind in a *qigong* state.

Movements:

a. Stand with the feet apart to shoulder width, and bend the legs slightly.

b. Keep the head and neck upright, draw the chest in, relax the shoulders, drop the hands naturally, open the armpits slightly and relax your entire body.

c. Close the eyes slightly.

d. Breathe naturally and evenly.

Breathing adjustment:

Adjust your breathing after repeating each character six times.

Movements:

a. Raise the arms slowly upward from both sides to a level slightly below the shoulders, palms downward.

b. Turn the palms over with the elbows as the axis, palms upward.

c. Bend the elbows and draw circles inward with the forearms.

d. Keep the fingers opposite each other and in front of the chest, move them to the abdomen gradually with the palms downward, and then bring them down to the sides and return to the starting form, breathe naturally.

[1] Xu (like the word "you" in scottish pronunciation) (Fig. 12-87)

Mouth form: Close the lips slightly and stick the tongue forward and roll both sides of the tongue inward slightly.

Effect: This has a curative effect for eye trouble, the decline of liver functions, poor appetite, and dizziness.

Movements:

a. Put one hand on top of the other below the navel (the Dantian acupoint), left hand under for men and right hand under for women.

b. Touch the big toes to the ground lightly, stare, produce the sound of "xu" while contracting on the abdomen and breathing out.

c. Breathe in naturally after the stale air is totally exhaled. Do this 6 times.

The line of the movement for mental activity: Move the mental energy along the following channels and collaterals of the meridian system while doing the exercise: The outer side of the big toes → insteps → the inner side of the knees → perineum → the lower abdomen → the liver → the chest → the back of the throat → the eyes and brain.

[2] He (like the word "her") (Figs. 12-88, 12-89)

Mouth form: Keep the mouth half open, and stick the tongue against the lower palate.

Effect: This has a curative effect for palpitations, heart disease, insomnia, amnesia, night sweats and tongue ulcers.

Movements:

a. The same movements as those in a. b. c. in the above-mentioned "breathing adjustment." Keep the fingers opposite each other and in front of the chest.

b. Move the hands downward after touching the big toes to the ground, and at the same time open the mouth wide to pronounce "he," and breathe out. Breathe out totally when the hands reach the lower abdomen. Do this 6 times.

The line of movement for mental activity: The inner side of the big toes→the inner side of the legs→the abdomen→the spleen and stomach→the chest→the heart→the brain.

[3] Hu (Figs. 12-90, 12-91)

Mouth form: Pout the lips and stick the tongue forward energetically to drive out *qi* from the internal thoroughfare vessel to let it gush out of the mouth.

Effect: This has a curative effect for weak spleen, indigestion, spleen and stomach disorder, atrophy of the sinews and muscles, bleeding stool, and menstrual disorders.

Movements:

a. Position your hands as though holding something between them, palms upward, and move them up from the abdomen to the chest.

b. Rotate the wrists, palms outward.

c. Touch the big toes to the ground, move the right palm to the upper right and the left palm to the lower left, and at the same time breathe out with the sound of "hu."

d. Turn the palms over after exhaling totally, then inhale, move the right hand downward from the upper right and the left hand upward from the lower left to meet in front of the chest.

e. Turn both hands over with the palms outward, begin to do the second "hu" cycle of movements, and move the left hand to the upper left and the right hand to the lower right.

f. After the c. d. e. movements are done alternately, 3 times each, the hands meet in front of the chest, palms downward, and

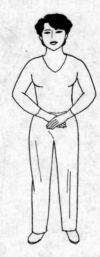

Fig. 12-87

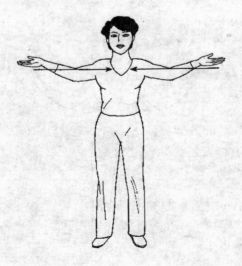

Fig. 12-88

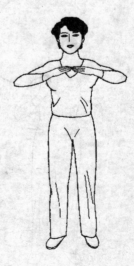

Fig. 12-89

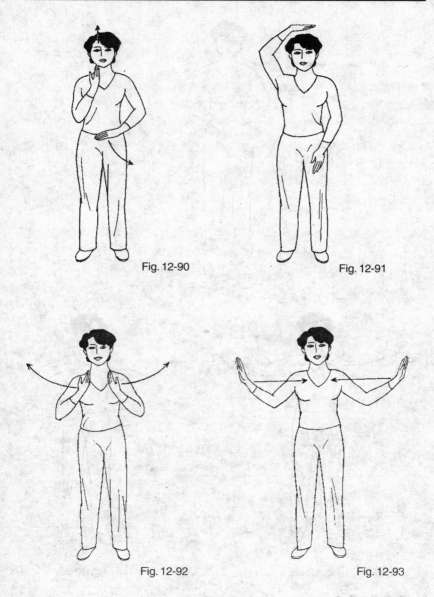

Fig. 12-90

Fig. 12-91

Fig. 12-92

Fig. 12-93

then move to the abdomen and return to the starting position.

The line of movement for mental activity: The inner side of the big toes→the inner side of the legs→the abdomen→the stomach →under the tongue.

[4] Si (like the "s" in study, long drawn out) (Figs. 12-92, 12-93)

Mouth form: Draw back the lips slightly, close the upper and lower teeth, and stick the tip of the tongue against them to pronounce the sound "si."

Effect: This has a curative effect for colds, coughs, shortness of breath, frequent urination, sore back, and pulmonary tuberculosis.

Movements:

a. Position your hands as though holding something, and move them from the abdomen up to the chest.

b. Keep the palms outward and fingers upward.

c. Touch the big toes to the ground, produce the sound "si" and exhale, with the arms apart on both sides.

d. Breathe all the *qi* out after moving the arms apart to the sides.

e. Drop the arms down naturally and return to the starting position.

The line of movement for mental activity: The outer side of the big toes → the insteps → the inner side of the legs → the large intestine → the stomach → the lungs → under the armpits → the inner side of the arms→the thumbs.

[5] Chui (like the word "tree", with the "r" pronounced as a "ue") (Fig. 12-94, 12-95)

Mouth form: The mouth looks closed, but is actually not, the corners of the mouth are slightly contracted inward, and the tongue is stuck forward, but slightly contracted.

Effect: This has a curative effect for lumbago, sore feet, dry eyes, amnesia, night sweats, dizziness, emission and hair loss.

Movements:

a. Put the backs of the hands against the back part of the waist.

b. Move the hands from the waist upward to under the armpits, and stretch them forward from both sides to before the chest, as if holding a ball, fingers of both hands opposite each other.

c. Touch the toes of both feet to the ground, breathe out while squatting downward, and pronounce the sound of "chui."

d. Move the arms downward while squatting down, with the hands reaching the knees at the end of the exhalation.

e. Stand up slowly, and keep the arms down by the sides.

The line of movement for mental activity: The soles→the inner ankle bones→the inner side of the shanks→the inner side of the thighs→the coccyx→the kidneys→the abdomen→the heart→ under the armpits→the inner side of the arms→the tips of the middle fingers.

[6] Xi (like the word "see") (Figs. 12-96, 12-97, 12-98, 12-99)

Mouth form: Open the lips slightly and slightly inward, and stick the tongue flat out, but shrink it slightly.

Effect: This has a curative effect for tinnitus, dizziness, sore throat, oppressive feeling in the chest, abdominal distention and urinary disorders.

Movements:

a. Smile.

b. Position the hands as though propping something up, and move them from the sides of the body to the pubic bones.

c. Keep the fingers opposite each other, and move them up to the chest.

d. Turn the wrists outward, palms outward.

e. Touch the fourth and fifth toes of both feet to the ground and pronounce the sound of "xi," and exhale.

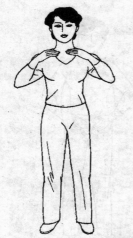

Fig. 12-94

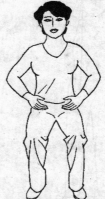

Fig. 12-95

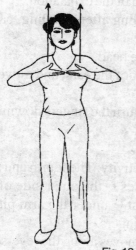

Fig. 12-96

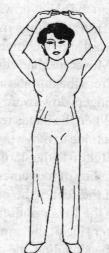

Fig. 12-97

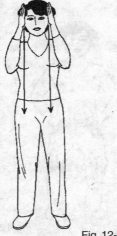 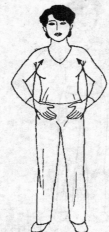

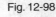
Fig. 12-98   Fig. 12-99

f. Lift the hands upward until the end of the exhalation.

g. Turn the palms over while inhaling after exhaling, palms downward and five fingers apart.

h. Move the hands downward to the head.

i. Press the thumbs against the back of the ears, and move the other fingers downward on the cheeks.

j. When the hands reach the chest, turn the fingers downward and continue to move them to the sides.

k. Return to the starting position.

The line of movement for mental activity: The fourth and fifth toes of the feet → the outer ankle bones → the outer side of the legs → the lower abdomen → the chest → under the arm pits → the outer side of the arms → the index fingers.

When inhaling, the mental energy moves along the reverse direction of the same line: the ring fingers → the outer side of the arms

→ the shoulders → the back side of the ears → the sides of the body→the outer side of the legs→the fourth toes.

Adjust your breathing after finishing the six-character-formula. Now, the entire exercise is completed. The effect will be even better if you now stand in silence for 7-8 minutes in the starting form.

It is not difficult to learn to do the six-character formula well, but the key to it is to grasp the following essential points:

[1] Begin by dispelling all distracting thoughts. After you stand in silence for a few minutes, an electric current seems to flow past inside of your body. The effect is especially good if you begin the exercise at this point.

[2] Grasp the breathing method well, contract the abdomen when you inhale, and extend the abdomen when you exhale. A special feature of the six-character formula is that you first exhale and then inhale, and breathe out while producing the sounds, and at the same time contract the anus and kidneys, and then take in fresh air.

[3] Pronounce the sounds accurately, because every sound is linked with a corresponding channel of the meridian system. Therefore, accurate pronunciation is essential. At the beginning, you must produce the sound. After you practise it long enough and get used to it, you may just exhale and mouth the word without actually producing the sound.

[4] Shift the body weight backward when you practise this exercise. Begin to exhale immediately after you touch the toes to the ground. At the same time, the body weight should be gradually shifted backward to the heels, the toes and soles slightly off the ground.

[5] You must use the mind to guide the flow of *qi*. The mental activity and the exhalation should start at the same time. Without this mental activity, the effect of *qigong* is quite different. Therefore, remember the line of movement for mental activity and use the mind to guide the flow of *qi*.

[6] Open your eyes wide when you do the "xu" character exercise. If you have a slight pain in the eyeballs as if they are pierced by a needle, just do not be scared. Because it is the effect of the *qigong*. Your eyes will be very bright after you practise it for some time.

[7] Do the exercise with perseverance, twice a day, 30 minutes each time. You will see results in 10 days.

(14) Mawangdui Daoyin physical and breathing exercise

The No. 3 Tomb of the Han Dynasty (206 BC-AD 220) at Mawangdui was unearthed in Changsha, Hunan Province in central China in 1973. Among the relics in the tomb was a color silk painting *Daoyin Diagram*, 140 cm long, 100 cm wide and 50 cm high. In this painting, 44 figures of different types are practising various kinds of exercises. This portrays the essence of the Daoyin method for health preservation in ancient China.

The Daoyin method stimulates the function of *qi* (vital energy) and promotes the primordial energy in the body to clear the cerebrum of bad information through exercise and regulation. The painting in Changsha shows both the dynamic and static methods, or a combination of the two. Some people are doing physical and breathing exercises, and some are doing exercises using various apparatuses. Most conspicuously, many are doing exercises in imitation of animal movements.

People have since worked out a set of "Mawangdui Daoyin health exercises" based on this Changsha painting.

The Daoyin exercise may be summed up as "concentrate the mind on two things," namely, one a good idea, and the other a complete circulation circle of *qi* throughout the body. It is said that as long as you do the exercise calmly and concentrate your mind as required, you will become apparently tipsy, but not actually tipsy, and may even dance along as if in the rosy clouds for the first time. People have different degrees of feelings after doing it for a few days. They may feel warm, cool, light, heavy, large, small, itchy or numb and it can have different effects on different diseases.

This exercise has certain curative effects for chronic diseases and difficult cases, especially conditions caused by endocrinopathy, cardiovascular diseases and diseases of the motor and respiratory systems.

The Daoyin exercise consists of seven steps and is done as described in the following:

Step One: Sit in silence with concentrated attention (or stand or lie).

This requires the practitioners to discharge both stool and urine, loosen clothing, unfasten belts, and refrain from smoking, drinking alcohol or eating pungent food. A large, safe, airy and quiet spot should be chosen in which to exercise. The best time to practise is between 5 and 7 in the morning or between 8 and 11 in the evening. Keep calm and concentrate your mind. Whether in the sitting or lying position, place your hands on the Dantian region (the left hand under for men and the right hand under for women), and stick the tongue against the upper palate. In the standing position, drop the shoulders and elbows, draw in the chest, straighten the back and keep the palms opposite each other as if embracing a large tree. Think out a good idea and breathe naturally. Relax the muscles as much as possible so there are no disquieting thoughts in your mind. To achieve all this, first adjust the body posture and breathing, and then count the number of breaths from one to nine until there is not a single distracting thought in your mind. At the same time, close the seven apertures of the head as tightly as possible to hear your own breathing sounds. When you can hear your breathing, concentrate your mind on Dantian, Mingmen and Baihui, or Dantian, Mingmen and Huiyin (for diseases below Dantian) so that the exercise goes round and begins again three times to form a simple complete circulation cycle of *qi*.

Step Two: Complete circulation cycle of *qi*.

A complete circulation cycle of *qi* uses the mind to guide the circulation of *qi* and blood in a complete circle throughout the body. This requires you to stick your tongue against the upper palate and imagine that a mass of *qi* and blood is passing through the Huiyin acupoint. Contract the anus and the anal muscles at this time. When you feel the flow of *qi* at Huiyin, guide the *qi* circulatiion to the coccyx, Mingmen, Jiaji, Dazhui, Yuzhen, and Baihui, and make a circle over the Baihui acupoint on the top of the head (clockwise for men and counterclockwise for women), and then from Baihui to Zuqiao, Queqiao, Laogong, Chonglou, Danzhong, Dantian, Huiyin and Yongquan. Repeat the cycle three times, and concentrate the mind on Dantian during the last cycle. (Fig. 12-100)

Step Three: Swing the heavenly column (cervical vertebra) slightly.

After a slight pause, begin to practise the exercise of swinging the cervical vertebra. This requires you to continue concentrating the mind on Dantian, and look to the right and to the left like a white crane looking for food, or as though swinging with a ball from right to left. Turn the hands and the body slowly to the left and right together with the cervical vertebra. Raise the right hand slowly to the Baihui acupoint on the top of the head and change it into a palm facing downward. Move the left hand to Dantian and change it into a palm facing upward. Then turn the trunk slowly from right to left. Repeat the exercise 9 times.

Step Four: Imagine a snow fountain.

Imagine a mass of snow in the heat and a fountain of warm water in the cold washing down from the Baihui acupoint at the top of the head, past the face, the arms, Danzhong, Dantian and Huiyin to Yongquan and the tips of the toes. Imagine this three times.

Step Five: Read a pithy saying in silence.

Imagine it is springtime with bright sunshine and a gentle breeze, and you are in a quiet place with flowers in full bloom, birds singing, and your body is moving slightly like the willow in the breeze. At the same time, imagine the meaning of the saying: "All worries disappear in the midnight silence, the whole body is relaxed and soft and sways with the wind. Concentrate on Dantian and close all apertures of the head, and feel happy and pleased as if flying into the sky." Now, your mind is at ease. Your whole body is relaxed and soft, and feels light, as light as if it were flying to the moon and roaming the skies.

Step Six: Keep the body weight on the heels and do not try to control them. If they want to move, let them move; if they want to fly, let them fly. If they do not move, let them stay like that, relaxed and free.

Step Seven: Wind up the exercise.

Begin to wind up the exercise after practising it for 30-60 minutes. Just concentrate the mind on the Yongquan acupoint (the left for men and the right for women), and say in silence repeatedly: "I want to wind up the exercise. I want to stop." If you cannot stop, just open your eyes and have a look. When the body becomes firm, begin to raise your hands from the buttocks and join them at Dantian, upward to the chest, around the ears, and finally massage the Baihui point 9 times. For the massage, keep the left hand under the right hand for men and move them clockwise, and the right hand under the left hand for women, counterclockwise. Concentrate your mind on the tips of the middle fingers and let *qi* and blood rise and fall with the mental activity. Repeat 9 times.

When the massage is finished, rub the palms and the backs of the hands until they become warm, and then rub the cheeks and comb the hair 36 times in the order of the face, the top and back of the head. Finally walk slowly 30-50 steps and return *qi* to Dantian.

(15) Weight-reducing exercises

There are three weight-reducing exercises: The frog exercise, the lotus exercise, and the frog wave-stirring exercise.

The frog wave-stirring exercise helps most people alleviate or even get rid of their feeling of hunger. While practising this exercise, you should naturally reduce your eating, just eat a little vegetables and fruit. Generally, if you do not eat regular meals, you may feel dizzy, weak or suffer from low blood sugar, but this exercise helps reduce these adverse effects and you will not feel hungry. This shows that the weight-reducing *qigong* exercises help reduce your weight not only by cutting your diet, but by using its power to shift the nutrients to other parts of the body. Therefore, those doing this exercise use their surplus fat as energy to meet their daily needs.

[1] Frog exercise

a. Method: Posture: Sit upright in a chair 30-40 cm high, with feet on the ground, and keep the knees a part to shoulder width, the thighs and shanks forming angles of 90 degrees or a bit smaller. Put the elbows on the knees, clench one hand into a fist and hold the fist with the other (right hand fist for men and left hand fist for women). Bend the upper body forward, lower the head, and cushion the forehead with the fist eye. Close the eyes slightly and relax your whole body in a comfortable and natural posture. (Fig. 12-101)

Adjust mental activity: After taking the correct posture, both the mind and the nervous system enter into a state of relaxation and quiet. First draw a breath, and then you feel as if you are weak and limp, completely exhausted. Then, try to imagine the happiest and best thing in your life so that you become completely relaxed and cheerful in a minute or two.

Start the exercise: First concentrate the mind completely on breathing to avoid all outside interference, including noise. First draw a free breath into the abdomen, and then exhale it slowly through the mouth. While exhaling, relax your body and exhale it finely, slowly and evenly. The abdomen should become gradually soft and loose when the breath is exhaled. Draw another breath through the nose after exhaling, also finely, slowly and evenly. As the breath is being drawn, the abdomen expands gradually and finally becomes full. After the abdomen is full, stop breathing for two seconds, but keep yourself in a breathing state. Then draw a short breath. Exhale the air slowly right after the short breath. The breathing method is: Exhale-inhale-stop breathing for two seconds-short inhale, and repeat the cycle. Throughout the breathing process, the chest does not rise or fall, only the abdomen bulges and contracts like a frog expanding and contracting its abdomen when breathing.

Attention should be paid to the degree of fullness when drawing a breath which differs from person to person. Mind you, those who have bleeding internal organs or are recuperating from surgery must not practise this exercise. Cardiovascular disease sufferers or those with serious digestive system diseases should draw a breath for only one or two minutes. If a woman has heavier bleeding during her menstrual period after practising this exercise, she should just draw a breath for one, two, or three minutes, or simply stop practising it for the time being. If the menstrual period comes earlier than usual, she should also stop practising. Most people can breathe for eight or nine minutes. The breaths are drawn slowly and the abdomen becomes gradually full, and this is not a voluntary reaction of the abdominal muscles.

Wind up the exercise after doing it for 15 minutes. Do not open your eyes immediately or you may feel dizzy. Keep your eyes closed, raise your head slowly, raise your hands to the front of your chest, and rub your palms 10 times or more. Then comb your hair with your fingers several times before opening your eyes. After you open your eyes, clench the fists, stretch, and draw a deep and cool breath. By this time, your eyes will be bright and sharp and full of vigor.

b. Effect:

When inhaling, the abdominal pressure rises, forcing the blood of the internal organs to flow to the limbs and the head. When exhaling, the abdominal pressure obviously falls, and the blood in the limbs and the head flows back to the internal organs. This helps promote blood circulation throughout the body and produces a good effect on the body's metabolism. In turn, the improved metabolism and the increased flow of the blood help stimulate the circulation of the blood in the facial capillaries. This is excellent for skin care and hair growth.

The rise and fall of the diaphragm resulting from deep breathing also massages the internal organs, so it is helpful for the entire body, effectively promoting the transfer of internal energy and reducing or removing any harmful effects from a reduced diet.

While you are reducing weight, practise the exercise 3 times a day, about 15 minutes each time. You may practise either during mealtime or at any other time in a quiet place.

[2] Lotus exercise

a. Method:

Posture: The same as for the frog exercise, but you can sit with your legs crossed. When you sit, pile the hands, palms upward, and put them on the thighs. Keep the right hand above for men and the left hand above for women. Mind you, refrain from sitting against the back of the chair. Straighten the back slightly, draw in the chest and withdraw the chin. Stick your tongue lightly against the upper palate and close the eyes slightly, relax the eyebrows, and keep yourself comfortable and natural. (Fig. 12-102)

Adjust mental activity: After adjusting your posture, draw a full breath and relax. Then recall the happiest thing in your life for about

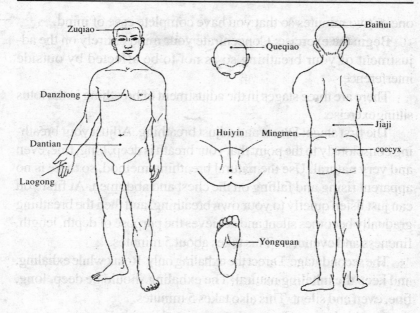

Fig. 12-100

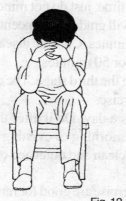

Fig. 12-101

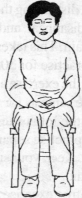

Fig. 12-102

one or two minutes so that you have complete ease of mind.

Begin the exercise: Concentrate your mind entirely on the adjustment of your breathing so as not to be affected by outside interference.

There are three stages in the adjustment of breathing in the lotus sitting exercise:

The first stage: Direct and adjust breathing. Adjust your breathing consciously to the point that your breath is deep, long, fine, even and very natural. Use the natural breathing method, so there is no apparent rising and falling on the chest and abdomen. At first you can just listen quietly to your own breathing, and then the breathing gradually becomes silent and achieves the purpose of depth, length, fineness and evenness. This takes about 5 minutes.

The second stage: Direct the exhaling only. Relax while exhaling, and keep the inhaling natural. The exhaling should be deep, long, fine, even and silent. This also takes 5 minutes.

The third stage: Change the consciously guided breathing to unconscious and natural breathing. This does not mean there is no conscious breathing since you always feel it faintly and continuously. If you have a distracting thought at this time, just do not mind it, but know it will disappear, and your mind will gradually concentrate on breathing again. This takes about 10 minutes. Chronic disease sufferers may practise for 30, or even 40 or 50 minutes.

Wind up the exercise after finishing the third stage. The closing method is the same as for the frog exercise.

Practise the lotus exercise 3 times a day. Do it after the frog exercise, or practise separately in the morning or evening before going to bed. Keep your surroundings clean and quiet and concentrate your mind.

Both the frog exercise and lotus exercise are good for removing fatigue, increasing metabolism, and treating many chronic diseases.

b. Effect:

The lotus exercise is mainly a simulation of genuine natural sleep. Generally speaking, people sleep for seven or eight hours a day, but genuine sleeping time is much shorter. Genuine sleep means complete relaxation of the body at rest. At this time, the cerebral cortex is completely inhibited. The third stage of breathing in this exercise is an imitation of genuine sleep in which the cerebral cortex approaches complete inhibition.

Therefore, the breathing in this exercise is divided into three stages. It helps to gradually develop from full consciousness to near-genuine sleep.

Practising these two exercises with good coordination helps to effectively counteract and alleviate the effects of a reduced diet.

[3] Frog wave-stirring exercise

a. Method:

Posture: Lie supine on the bed and bend the legs with the thighs and shanks forming an angle of 90 degrees. Keep both feet flat on the bed. Put one hand on the chest and the other on the belly, and begin to direct *qi*.

Start the exercise: Thrust out the chest and contract the abdomen (Fig. 12-103) when inhaling, and contract the chest and throw out the abdomen when exhaling. (Fig. 12-104) Protrude the abdomen as much as possible, but do not exert too much effort, as this may cause fatigue or strain. If you find something wrong with your chest or abdomen after this exercise, you should stop it for a few days.

As the chest and abdomen rise and fall like waves during the exercise, it is called the "frog wave-stirring exercise." Keep the breathing speed similar to regular breathing speed. If you breathe too quickly, you might feel dizzy. In that case, you should slow down the exercise.

It is worth noting that this exercise should be done only when you are hungry. The principle is "practise it whenever you are hungry, and do not practise when you are not hungry." Generally speaking, practise it before each meal everyday. If you are not hungry after the exercise, eat less or nothing at all. If you are hungry several times a day, practise it as soon as you feel hungry. When you have no hunger throughout the day, just stop doing it. Most people will lose the sense of hunger if they practise it 40 times a day. If you still feel hungry, practise 20 times more. If you are still hungry, please persist for one or two more days and the sense of hunger will become weak or disappear. Very few people will still have a strong sense of hunger after practising it 60 times a day. If this happens to you, stop doing it immediately.

The wave-stirring exercise can also be practised in the standing posture (Figs. 12-105, 12-106). Or you can do it while sitting, walking or even riding a bicycle.

b. Effect:

Why can the wave-stirring exercise eliminate the sense of hunger? This is not yet clear. At present, there are two reasons given:

The first says the sense of hunger is caused by the contraction of the empty stomach and the stimulation of the gastric mucous membrane by the gastric juice. This exercise is intended to force the gastric juice into the intestines through special breathing movement and the pushing and pressing movement of the stomach and intestines to greatly reduce the gastric juice, thus reducing its stimulation to the gastric mucous membrane. At the same time, because the movement of the chest and abdomen controls the contraction of the empty stomach, it helps eliminate hunger.

The other reason states that when hungry, the acidity of the digestive juice is distributed in trapezoid, it is more acid at places close to the gastric mucous membrane. This is why it causes hunger.

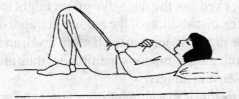

Fig. 12-103

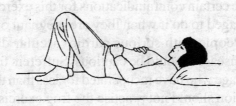

Fig. 12-104

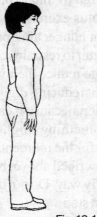 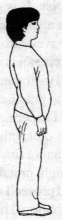

Fig. 12-105   Fig. 12-106

After practising exercise, the digestive juices might move up and down to upset the distribution of the acidity in trapezoid, weaken the acidity of the digestive juice at the bottom level, and reduce the stimulation to the gastric mucous membrane, thus alleviating or eliminating the sense of hunger.

What is interesting is that although the causes and principles are still under study, many people have alleviated or eliminated their sense of hunger after practising the exercise.

There are two remaining points for your attention:

a. There are certain contraindications for this exercise. Women are not encouraged to do it when they are pregnant or when they are nursing. People with serious cardiovascular diseases and enterogastric diseases should be cautious. Sufferers from internal organ hemorrhage who have recuperated for less than three months after an operation should not practise the frog exercises, but they can do the lotus exercise. You may increase the time for practising the exercise for reducing weight. Women can practise them as usual during the menstrual period. Do not inhale too much when you practise the frog exercise. It is good enough to inhale only 50 or 60 percent. They can also practise the lotus exercise more often. If some people still have a strong sense of hunger after practising the wave-stirring exercise and find it difficult to restrain it, they should stop practising and use other methods to reduce their weight.

b. If you want to practise the weight reducing *qigong* exercise, it is best to have an experienced teacher, because it calls for strict control over your diet, otherwise something might go wrong. However, if you cannot find a teacher for the moment, and are eager to try it, you might practise it as described above, but you must be very careful and proceed in an orderly way. Do not be impatient. Should anything abnormal happen, just stop.

Appendix:
Diagram of Acupoints of the Human Body

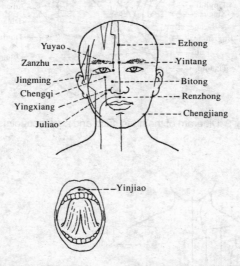

Fig. 1 Diagram of the head, face and neck acupoints (front)

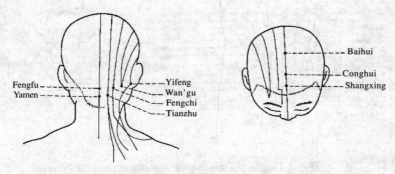

Fig. 2 Diagram of the head, face and neck acupoints (back)

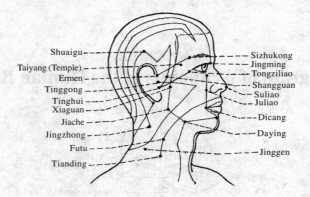

Fig. 3 Diagram of the head, face and neck acupoints (side)

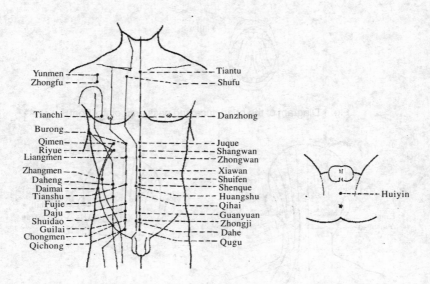

Fig. 4 Diagram of the chest and abdomen acupoints

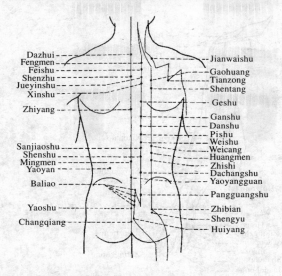

Fig. 5   Diagram of the back acupoints

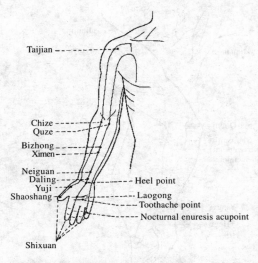

Fig 6   Diagram of the arm acupoints

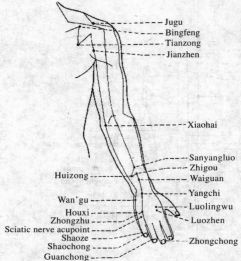

Fig. 7 Diagram of the arm acupoints

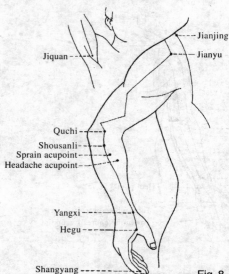

Fig. 8 Diagram of the arm acupoints

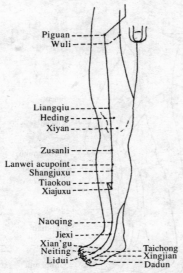

Piguan
Wuli
Liangqiu
Heding
Xiyan
Zusanli
Lanwei acupoint
Shangjuxu
Tiaokou
Xiajuxu
Naoqing
Jiexi
Xian'gu
Neiting
Lidui
Taichong
Xingjian
Dadun

Fig. 9   Diagram of the leg acupoints

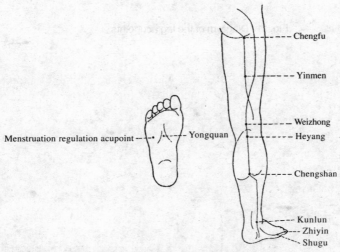

Chengfu

Yinmen

Weizhong
Heyang

Chengshan

Kunlun
Zhiyin
Shugu

Menstruation regulation acupoint
Yongquan

Fig. 10   Diagram of the leg acupoints

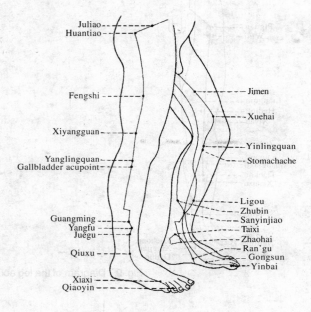

Fig. 11 Diagram of the leg acupoints